NOT YOUR ORDINARY COPING SKILLS BOOK

An Interactive and Customizable Guide to Being a Happier Adult

BY

Katie Parker MA, LPC

ACKNOWLEDGMENTS

This book is dedicated to ACT team D:

Dr. William McAllister, Randy Estes, Flo Williams, Dena Cochell, Brooke Sankiewicz, Kelly Bassham, Scott Price, Caarin Kogut, Gwen Williams, and Adam Hamilton. We were iconic and everything a team should be. I am a better person and therapist having learned from each of you.

A giant thank you to my incredible husband, Tom. If it weren't for your patience, support, and impressive graphic design skills, this book wouldn't exist.

To my beautiful daughter Nora, thank you for being you. You are my inspiration and the light of my life.

Thank you to my proof readers and wonderful parents, Debbie and Julian who always have my back.

To my colleagues Sharon Waldon and Dana Agrusa, thank you for your selfless willingness to help me grow.

Thank you to Kelly Brinkmann who always has me laughing with a funny story and a well-timed meme.

Finally, a special thank you to my life-long best friend Cari Stoller who always offers enthusiastic support. Our lengthy morale boosting venting sessions are the perfect coping skill.

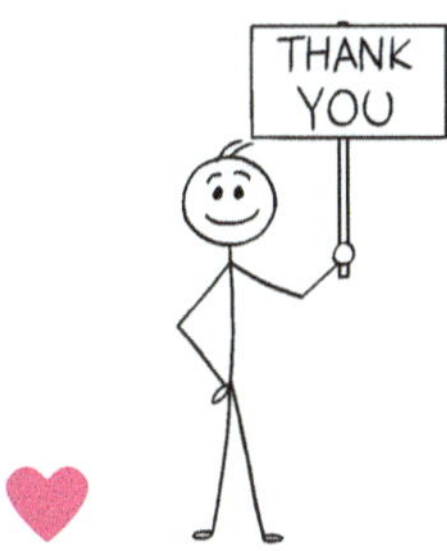

TABLE OF CONTENTS

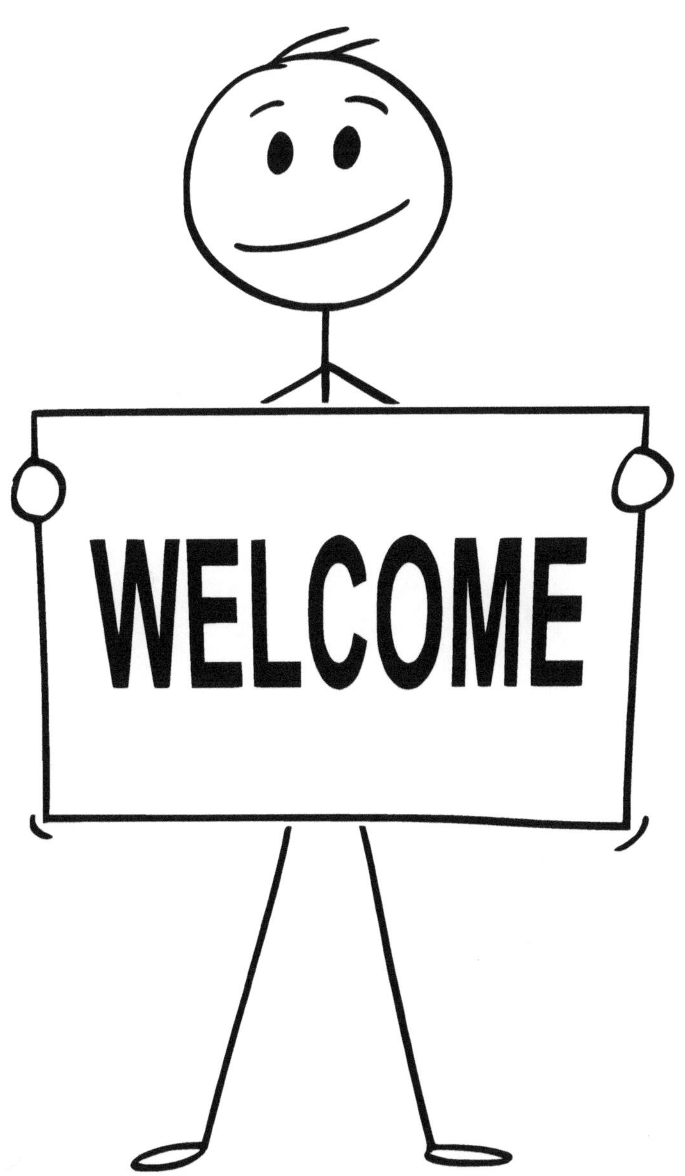
WELCOME

INTRODUCTION

Get excited! This book is an awesome hack to cope with life. By the time you reach the end of this book, you will have a whole new way of looking at coping skills. Plus, you will have created your own personalized coping skills toolkit! Consider this book your customized manual for effectively dealing with hard times throughout the rest of your life.

So, what makes this book different? It isn't just any ordinary therapy book about coping skills. This book is interactive and offers a fresh perspective by first organizing coping skills into six distinct categories. Toward the back, you will find a blank coping skills toolkit ready to be customized by you. As you brainstorm your personal coping strategies throughout each category, you will also jot them down in the corresponding section in the toolkit. There is even a bonus list of ideas and examples for each category provided at the back of the book for additional inspiration.

Feeling overwhelmed is a common experience and often leaves us struggling to come up with effective positive coping skills in the heat of the moment. It's as if our ability to think clearly takes a break, leaving us stranded. Imagine having a coping skills book bursting with strategies perfectly tailored to you, neatly organized into categories and ready to go! It'll be like having a secret weapon against stress and challenges, right at your fingertips. It will completely transform your approach to handling stress and adversity.

With the six-category method that I've created, it is easier to match an appropriate coping skill to the intensity of the problem. Being organized in this way allows you to look in each category to find an assortment of options you might not have otherwise considered. After you have read through all six categories, you'll have opened your mind to a greater world of coping possibilities and created an effective coping skills collection just for you!

Where did the six categories come from? Throughout the years in my therapy practice, I've had the chance to guide many in reshaping how they deal with stress and tough emotions by building up their own unique set of coping tools. Since coping skills are not universal, what works for me might not necessarily work for you, I found it important to have each individual create their own tailor-made list. I also noticed something else. When I neatly organized coping skills into categories, people seemed to find more ways to effectively cope and would brainstorm way more efficiently. Over time, as I honed the method, I found that positive coping skills seemed to naturally fall into six categories.

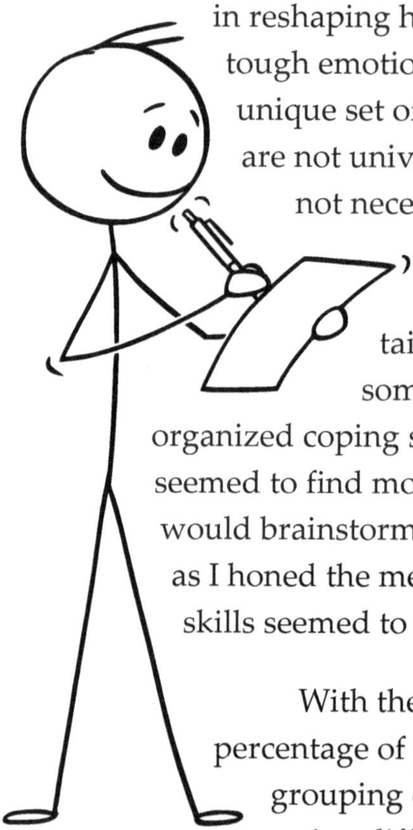

With the knowledge that a large percentage of people are better visual learners, grouping coping strategies together and using different colors for each category was a game-changer. Having a visually pleasing and organized physical list that you could continue to add to, took it from a therapeutic conversation to an actual useful tool. The ultimate tool really, because it's like giving yourself a detailed and color-coded plan to navigate through tough times.

The aim here is to build a lengthy list over time. Think of it like building a diverse menu or stocking up a toolbox – the more options you have in each category, the better equipped you'll be to handle whatever life throws your way. Keep adding to your list throughout the years and watch it grow!

Ultimately, my goal in creating this book is to empower individuals like yourself to take charge of your mental well-being and equip you with the necessary tools to navigate life's challenges.

There are certain interventions routinely used in therapy that are consistently effective and provide relief for many types of symptoms, diagnoses, and problems. I am excited to share these coping skills with you. I know that by developing and practicing positive coping skills, you can have a happier life, so let's get started!

Chapter 1 Coping Skills

What Are Coping Skills?

First, let's start by defining what a coping skill is, so that we are sure to be on the same page. You will not actually find this term in the most popular dictionaries, although the term is widely known and commonly used in the mental health field. Coping skills (also sometimes referred to as coping strategies, coping tools, coping techniques or coping mechanisms) are methods used to help relieve discomfort associated with difficult emotions, stress, and symptoms.

When people are faced with difficult situations, they typically develop or use coping mechanisms to deal with the stress and emotions that arise. Positive coping skills provide us with healthy ways to manage and reduce stress. When we have effective coping skills, we are better equipped to handle the challenges and pressures that life throws at us.

However, not all coping mechanisms are healthy or beneficial. Negative coping skills such as substance abuse or excessive eating may provide temporary relief, although in the long run, there is potential for risk and consequence and can make problems worse or create new issues.

By learning more about coping strategies, you can leverage the information to compile your own list of positive coping skills and replace any negative coping skills you may have with healthier alternatives helping to successfully improve your ability to overcome life's challenges and reduce emotional discomfort.

Negative Coping Skills

Before we continue, let's take a moment to talk a little more about negative coping skills. Negative coping can include unhealthy habits or behaviors that provide instant relief fooling you into believing that they are a reasonable option. However, these deceptive strategies might compound the problem or create new issues.

One common example is substance use. Turning to alcohol, drugs, or even over the counter medication to numb your feelings or escape from reality can be a bad gamble. While it might provide a temporary escape, it could actually make you feel worse after the immediate effect wears off and can seriously impact your physical and mental health. Medication can absolutely be a valuable tool when prescribed by a medical professional and managed properly. Speaking with a medical provider who can properly diagnose and treat can find the right medication to help reduce or eliminate symptoms.

While it might seem helpful to numb the pain or escape from reality, relying on negative coping skills can actually bring on additional trouble. When you turn to unhealthy ways to cope with stress or difficult emotions, you're essentially putting a Band-Aid on a much bigger wound. Sure, it might dull the ache for a little while, but it doesn't actually fix whatever is causing the pain in the first place.

Plus, there's the whole slippery slope thing to consider. Whether the unhealthy coping mechanism is substance use, overeating, excessive spending, etc., the cost can soon outweigh the temporary benefit by taking a potential toll not just on your mental and physical health, but also your finances, employment and relationships.

The thing to remember is that negative coping skills might feel good in the moment, but they rarely help you in the long term. It's important to recognize when you're falling into these patterns and try to find healthier ways to cope, including reaching out for support and seeking professional help when needed.

Spin the wheel on this scenario! Your friend, the character that he is, with a penchant for excitement, finds himself in a bit of a pickle after a particularly stressful week. Instead of unwinding with a mindfulness activity like yoga or a self-soothing hot sauna, he decides to roll the dice and distract himself by hitting the casino floor. The flashing lights, the rhythmic chime of slot machines, it's all too tempting to resist. He throws caution to the wind and starts betting with the enthusiasm of someone who just discovered the concept of "beginner's luck." As the chips start to stack against him, his heart races and he starts to have an upset stomach. When the dust settles and his wallet is emptier than a bird feeder during a squirrel convention, he realizes he's played a risky game with more consequences than he bargained for. It's like trying to find treasure in a

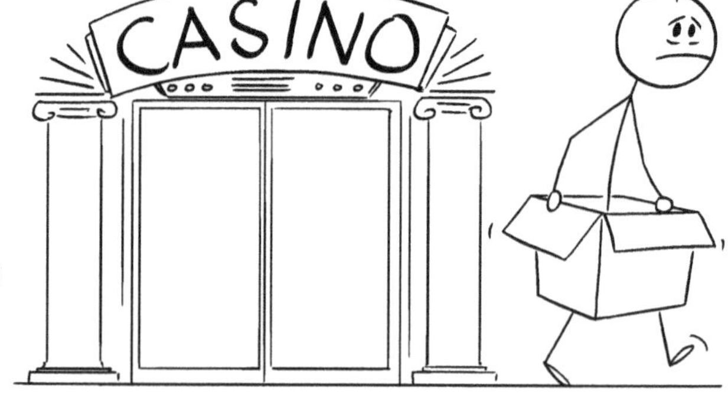

minefield—sure, there might be some shiny moments, but the explosions of regret are bound to follow!

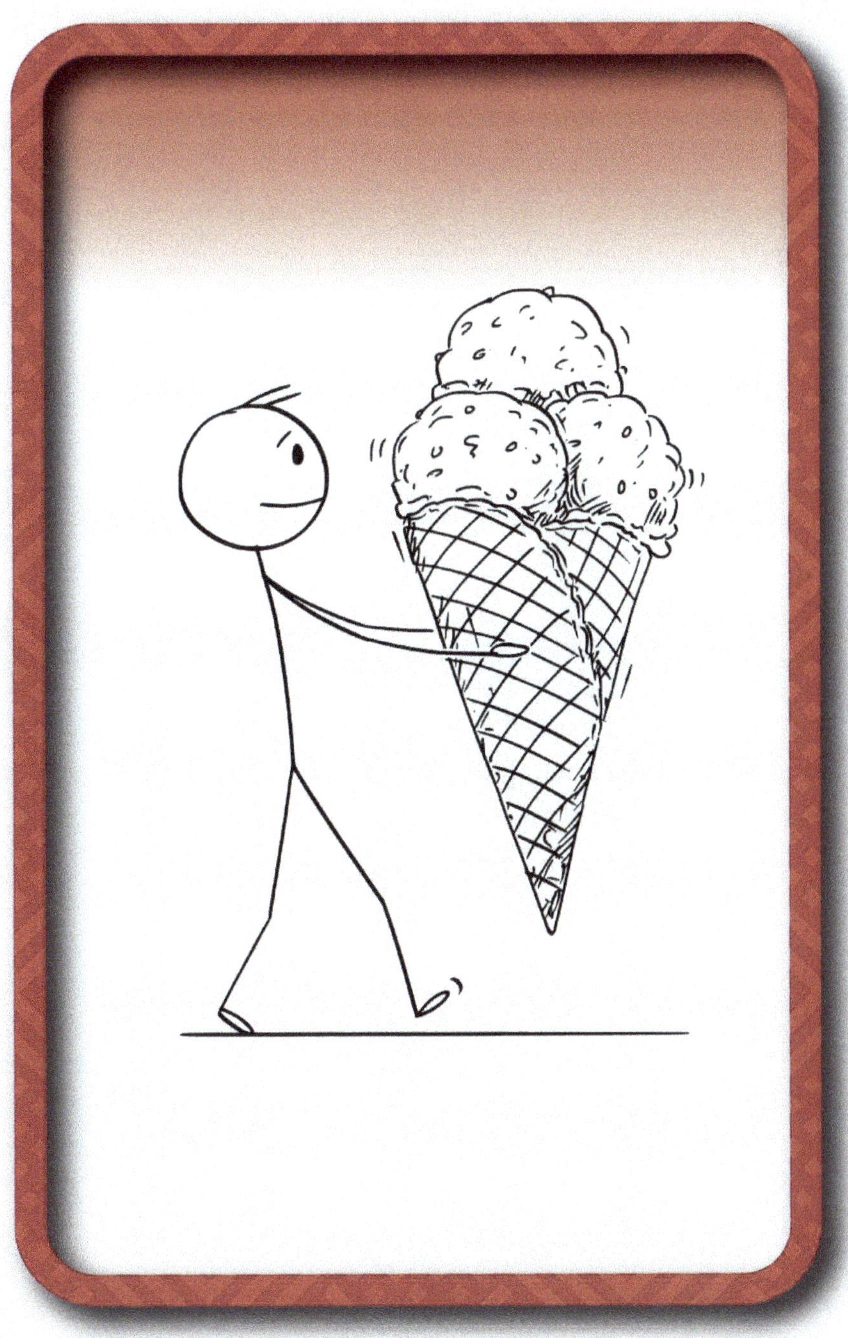

Sample List

Negative Coping

Avoidance

Substance use

Procrastination

Emotional overeating

Oversleeping

Self-harm

Aggression

Withdrawing/Isolating

Seeking constant validation

Engaging in risky behaviors

Overspending

Blame

People pleasing

Emotional detachment

Suppressing emotions

Gambling

Self-deprecating

Plotting revenge

Are there any negative coping skills that you currently use or have used in the past?

____

____

____

____

____

Positive Coping Skills

Now that we are more aware of our potential pitfalls, we can turn our attention to positive coping. In my years of experience as a therapist, I have witnessed the transformative power of effective and healthy coping. Positive coping skills are not just temporary fixes; they are valuable tools that you can carry throughout your life. The more you have, the better!

When you have a large number of effective coping skills to choose from, you gain greater ability to reduce the intensity and more quickly deescalate stress, regulate emotions, and navigate challenging situations. Having effective means of coping enables you to take control of your life with greater ease even in the face of adversity.

Compiling a full list of ready to use coping skills provides you with a sense of empowerment and control. As you become more proficient in using these skills, you gain confidence in your ability to handle difficult emotions and situations. This confidence can have a ripple effect, positively impacting various areas of your life. Through consistent use of diverse types of positive coping skills in your daily life, you can enhance your overall quality of life and be able to decrease the impact of uncomfortable emotions.

Having positive effective coping skills helps with emotional regulation. Regulating your own emotions improves ability to express feelings in a healthy manner, prevents emotional outbursts and averts physical impact such as changes in appetite or sleep disturbance. When you have strong emotional regulation skills, you can navigate through difficult situations without becoming overwhelmed by your emotions. You can recognize and acknowledge your emotions without letting them control you. Coping skills can help you regulate your emotions and maintain emotional balance.

Positive coping skills build resilience, which is the ability to bounce back from adversity. They help you navigate through challenging situations and come out stronger on the other side. When you face setbacks or obstacles, having many healthy coping skills to choose from allows you to better adapt and persevere.

Developing a long list of effective and healthy coping mechanisms also helps you to problem-solve, think critically, and maintain a positive mindset. It provides you with the tools to overcome obstacles, have flexible and adaptive thinking and use strategy. Essentially it can help you get unstuck and move forward.

Using positive coping skills is an act of self-care. It shows that you prioritize your well-being and take proactive steps to maintain your mental and emotional health. By learning how to turn down the intensity or resolve distress, you are investing in your overall mental health. Taking the time to create a personalized positive coping skills list tailored to your specific needs and preferences is the ultimate way to be prepared for whatever life throws your way.

Everyone Is Unique

While there are numerous coping skills available, it's important to find the positive ones that work best for you. The things that help me to cope might aggravate you. So, the key is to identify what works for you and what helps you cope with stress and difficult emotions.

Also, it is important to note that sometimes your go-to coping skill will not always work every time or in every situation, which is why you need an extensive list of alternative coping strategies. The brainstorm list of possible coping skills ideas you will find at the back of this book will help to get you thinking about different ways to cope and by putting them into six categories, you'll think about using them in a whole new way.

Here are some tips to consider when developing your own customized coping skills toolkit:

EXPERIMENTATION: Try out different coping skills to see what resonates with you. Explore what works in different settings. Try different coping skills in various environments to identify where a coping skill might not work and try an alternative. The important thing is to experiment and find what brings you relief and helps you to deescalate.

BE OPEN TO CHANGE: Coping skills can evolve over time, so it's important to remain open to trying new strategies. As you grow and change, your coping skills may need to adapt as well. What worked for you in the past may not work as effectively now, and that's okay.

Be willing to explore new coping mechanisms and be open to adjusting your approach as needed. Remember, coping is a lifelong process, and it's important to be flexible and patient in finding what works best for you.

IDENTIFY YOUR TRIGGERS: **Understand what situations,** thoughts, or emotions tend to trigger stress, anxiety, or other negative feelings for you. By recognizing your triggers, you can tailor your coping strategies to address them more effectively. For example, if public speaking causes anxiety, you can include techniques like deep breathing or visualization in your toolkit to manage that specific trigger. (You went right to thinking of people in their underwear, didn't you?)

PRACTICE CONSISTENTLY: **Consistency is important when it** comes to developing coping skills. You will want to regularly use and practice the techniques you've chosen for your toolkit, even when you're not feeling particularly stressed. This will help you become more proficient at using them and integrate them into your daily routine. Additionally, practicing your coping skills proactively can help build cognitive pathways, making it easier to cope when you encounter similar stressful situations in the future.

SEEK PROFESSIONAL GUIDANCE: **If you're unsure where to** start or need additional support, consider reaching out to a therapist. They can provide guidance and help you explore coping skills that align with your specific needs and goals. A counselor can help you identify any underlying issues that may be contributing to your emotional distress and provide you with additional tools and strategies to manage them effectively.

By engaging in self-reflection, experimenting with different coping skills, seeking professional guidance, and being open to change, you can find the coping skills that are most effective for you.

Remember, everyone is different, and what works for someone else may not work for you. It's important to find the coping skills that resonate with your unique personality and help you navigate the challenges and stressors of life in a healthy and productive way.

Using the Right Tools

So, when should you whip out those coping skills? Well, the short answer is: whenever you need them! But let's break it down a bit more. We've discussed that coping skills are like tools in a toolbox. There are different tools to use, each one designed for different situations. Just like you wouldn't use a hammer to tighten a screw, you want to match the coping skill to the level of distress you're experiencing.

Let's say you're feeling a bit stressed out because of a looming deadline at work. In this case, you might reach for a self-soothing technique like taking a luxurious bubble bath and also use a positive self-talk skill such as confidence building affirmations to help take the edge off. These skills are perfect for mild to moderate levels of distress and can help you regain a sense of calm and focus.

Now, let's kick it up a notch. Imagine, out of nowhere you all of a sudden find yourself having a full-blown panic attack. Your heart is racing, your palms are sweaty, and it feels like the world is closing in around you. In situations like these, grounding techniques can be a real lifesaver. As a mindfulness skill, grounding techniques such as using your five senses to observe your surroundings, can help bring you back to the present moment and provide some much-needed relief.

Imagine you're feeling angry because someone cut in front of you in line at the grocery store. Instead of blowing your top, you take a deep breath and repeat to yourself that getting angry won't change the situation. This is an example of using self-soothing and positive self-talk coping skills to calm down when you're feeling heated. If further coping is needed, you can mentally scan through each of the six categories we will soon discuss and see if there are better coping tools to use.

But here's the cool part: the more you practice using different coping skills, the easier it becomes to choose the right one for each situation. It's like building a muscle – the more you work it out, the stronger it gets. Eventually, you'll find that coping skills become second nature, and you'll instinctively know which one to use based on how you're feeling.

By matching the coping skill to the level of distress you're experiencing, you can effectively manage your emotions and navigate even the trickiest of situations. So go ahead, keep reading so we can learn a helpful way to gauge your level of distress in order to make best use of your own amazing coping skills toolkit that you will soon develop. You've got this!

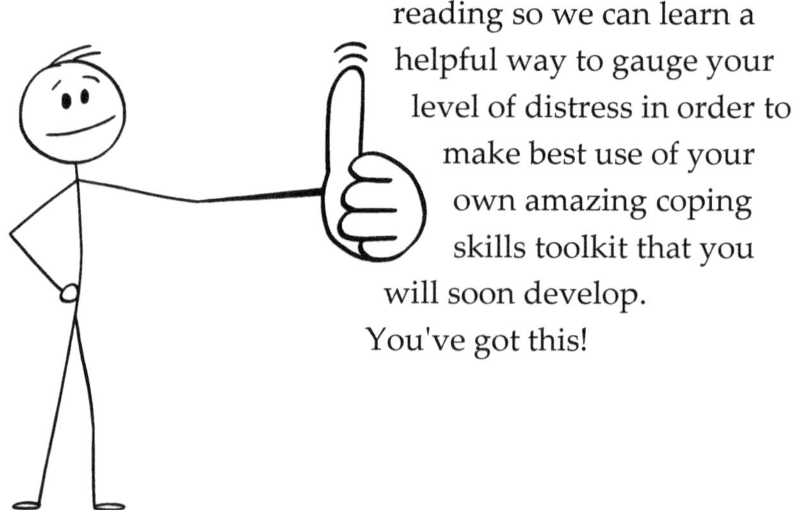

Chapter 2 Distress Thermometer

Visualizing Your Distress Thermometer

Okay, so how do I decide which coping skill to use? Well, one important factor is evaluating how upset you are. To do this, may I suggest using visualization to gauge your level of distress. Picture this: a thermometer with numbers ranging from 1 to 10, where 10 represents the most distressed you can possibly feel.

Now, you might be wondering, "Why visualize a thermometer?" Well, it's a handy way to check in with yourself and get a clear picture of how you're feeling. Just like checking the weather forecast before heading out, knowing your distress level can help you prepare and take appropriate action to manage your emotions.

Let me share a personal story to demonstrate this. Recently, at the start of vacation, my picture ID mysteriously went missing at the airport during bag check and before I went through security. My anxiety and worry were through the roof. I was nervous that I would not be allowed to travel and would have to cancel my trip to Florida.

I checked in with myself and knew I was hovering around a 9 on the distress thermometer. Once I visualized it, I realized I needed to bring that number down to below an 8 before I could effectively problem solve. I took some deep breaths to soothe my central nervous system, and then when I was calm enough, I was able to find airport staff to ask for help.

Using Your Distress Thermometer

Now, let's break down how you can use this visualization technique in your own life:

VISUALIZE THE THERMOMETER: Close your eyes and imagine a thermometer in your mind. Picture the numbers 1 to 10 clearly marked on it, with 10 being the highest level of distress.

CHECK-IN WITH YOURSELF: Take a moment to assess how you're feeling. Are you feeling calm and collected like a 2 on the thermometer, or are you teetering closer to a 9 with overwhelming emotions?

BE HONEST WITH YOURSELF: It's essential to be honest about your feelings. Remember, there's no right or wrong level of distress. What matters is recognizing where you are on the scale and taking steps to address it.

IDENTIFY COPING STRATEGIES: Once you've pinpointed your distress level, think about what coping strategies might help you. If you're at a 3, maybe some distracting techniques could bring you down a notch. If you're at an 8, you might need more intensive techniques like asking for help.

BE REALISTIC: You cannot expect to go from a 10 to a zero. Instead, work toward deescalating and lowering the intensity. As the number lowers, your ability to better tolerate, cope and problem solve will increase.

MONITOR YOUR PROGRESS: As you implement coping strategies, keep an eye on your distress thermometer. Notice how your level of distress changes over time. Are your strategies helping you move down the scale? If not, don't be afraid to adjust and try something new.

PRACTICE SELF-COMPASSION: Remember, it's okay not to be okay sometimes. Be kind to yourself as you navigate your emotions. Give yourself some grace, patience and time.

So, the next time you're feeling overwhelmed, take a moment to visualize your distress thermometer. It's a simple yet effective tool for understanding and managing your emotions. And who knows, with a little practice, you might even become a pro at keeping your distress levels in check like me! I did make it to Florida after all.

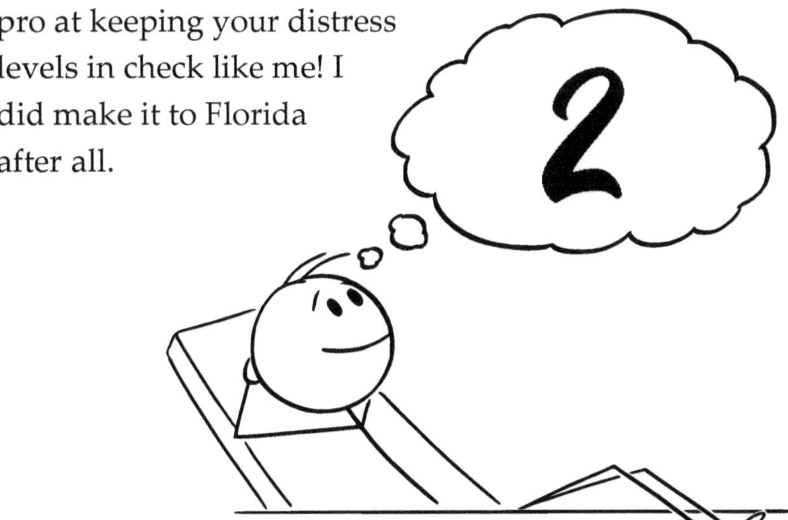

Your Very Own Distress Thermometer

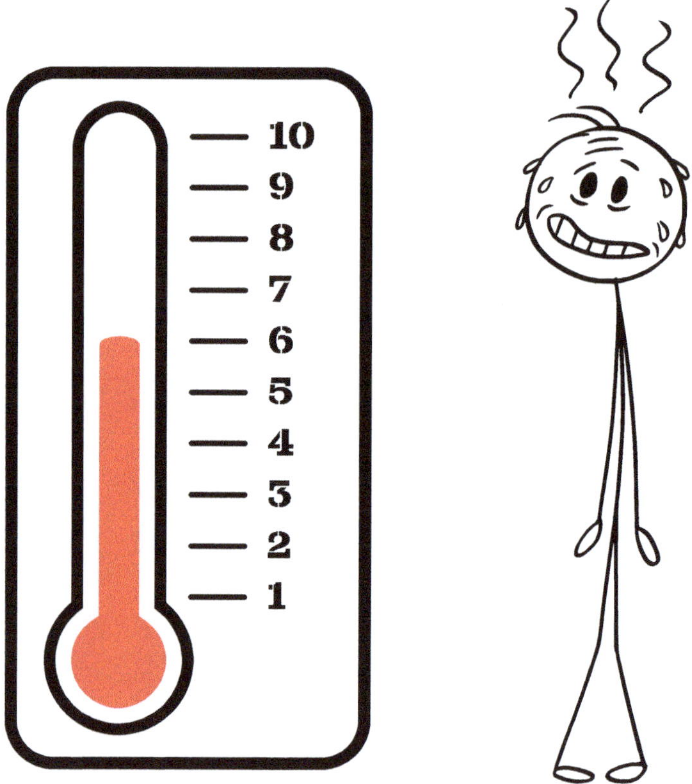

If your uncomfortable emotion or distress was a number 1-10 with 10 being the worst or most distressing and 0 being completely happy and calm which number would you be? Try to assign a number that correlates with the severity or intensity of your distress.

Chapter 3 Grey Area

Grey Area Coping Skills

Before I reveal the six categories of coping that I have been promising, it is important to know that there are certain coping skills that fall into sort of a grey area. I call these the "grey area" coping skills which can be positive if used in moderation, however, if overused can become negative coping skills with risk and consequence. Let's explore this nuanced territory in an attempt to understand what is helpful vs. harmful.

A Grey Area

We'll take a look at specific grey area coping skills, but first it's important to grasp why certain behaviors fall into this ambiguous category. Coping mechanisms, by nature, serve to alleviate stress or emotional discomfort. However, what distinguishes the grey area coping skills is their potential for misuse or over-reliance. While they may offer temporary relief, they can also foster dependency, create risk, and lead to negative consequences in the long run.

Below are some examples of potential grey area coping skills and should be evaluated and used with cost/risk/benefit mindset.

EATING: A dark chocolate square yes, a pint of chocolate ice cream, no. Research suggests that indulging in comfort foods can trigger the release of feel-good neurotransmitters like serotonin, temporarily lifting your mood.

Yet, relying on food as a self-soothing coping mechanism can lead to unhealthy eating patterns and weight gain. Emotional eating, characterized by consuming food in response to emotions rather than hunger, has been linked to obesity and other health issues. Therefore, while enjoying a favorite meal can offer solace, it's essential to cultivate a balanced relationship with food and practice moderation.

SHOPPING: **Sometimes hailed as "retail therapy,"** treating yourself at a store or making an online purchase can provide a fleeting sense of satisfaction, distracting from underlying stressors. Studies have shown that shopping can activate the brain's reward system, eliciting feelings of pleasure and gratification.

However, excessive shopping can lead to financial strain, debt, and clutter. Overspending as a coping mechanism may provide temporary relief and reward but can seriously exacerbate stress in the long term. It's crucial to differentiate between occasional and affordable indulgence and compulsive shopping tendencies.

ALCOHOL: **For some adults, relaxing with a glass of** wine at the end of a hectic day is a cherished ritual. Moderate alcohol consumption has been associated with relaxation and social bonding, thanks to its depressant effects on the central nervous system. In fact, studies suggest that moderate alcohol intake may have cardiovascular benefits and reduce the risk of certain diseases.

However, the line between moderate and excessive drinking can blur, especially when alcohol becomes a habitual coping mechanism. Relying on alcohol to cope with stress or negative emotions can lead to dependence, addiction, and a host of physical and mental health issues. It's essential to be mindful of reliance on alcohol consumption and explore alternative ways to unwind and manage stress.

SLEEP: Sleep is a great reset button, offering rejuvenation and restoration after a demanding day. Adequate sleep is necessary for cognitive function, mood regulation, memory retention and overall physical and mental wellness. During periods of stress, taking a 20-minute nap can provide temporary respite and recharge your battery so you can face things anew.

Yet, excessive sleeping or using sleep to avoid can indicate underlying issues such as depression or anxiety. Oversleeping may lead to lethargy, social withdrawal, and disruptions in daily routines. Sleeping during the day might mess with your circadian rhythm potentially causing insomnia at night. It's vital to address the root causes of sleep disturbances and adopt healthy sleep habits to ensure restorative rest.

SOCIAL MEDIA: In this digital age, social media has become a normal and often necessary part of daily life for people worldwide. Social media platforms offer the possibility for connection, self-expression, and information sharing. Engaging with social media can provide an online community of support, especially when feeling distressed or isolated.

Studies have shown that online social support can have positive effects on mental health, offering emotional validation and companionship.

Sadly, the constant exposure to curated images, status updates, and virtual comparisons on social media platforms can fuel feelings of inadequacy, jealousy, and FOMO (fear of missing out) which can contribute to decreased self-esteem and mood disturbance. Also, there is much misinformation spread online that can mistakenly be taken as fact.

The addictive nature of social media, including endless scrolling and compulsive checking, can exacerbate stress and distract from real-world coping strategies. Research suggests that excessive social media use may be associated with feelings of loneliness and mood disturbances including depression and anxiety, particularly among vulnerable populations such as adolescents and young adults.

Establishing boundaries around social media consumption, such as limiting screen time, curating a positive online environment, and engaging in meaningful interactions, can help mitigate its negative impact on mental health. Pay attention to your emotional reactions to social media and consider a digital detox or take breaks as needed.

SEX: Engaging in sexual activity is a natural and intimate way for adults to connect and experience pleasure. Sex can reduce stress, promote bonding between partners, and enhance mood through the release of oxytocin and endorphins. Sexual activity can be a form of positive coping, fostering emotional intimacy and physical satisfaction.

Nevertheless, relying on sex as a primary way to cope can pose risks, particularly when it involves risky behaviors or lacks emotional connection. Casual sex or compulsive sexual behavior driven by the need for validation or distraction from emotional distress can lead to negative consequences, including sexual health risks and relational conflicts.

Finding The Balance

Navigating the grey area of coping skills requires self-awareness and moderation. While these coping mechanisms may offer temporary relief at times, some are not sustainable solutions for managing stress and emotional challenges in the long term.

Grey area coping skills occupy a complex space in the realm of stress and mood management. While they may offer temporary relief and comfort, their overuse or misuse can lead to negative consequences. By considering the nuances and cultivating a balanced approach, you can navigate challenges and side-step potential issues.

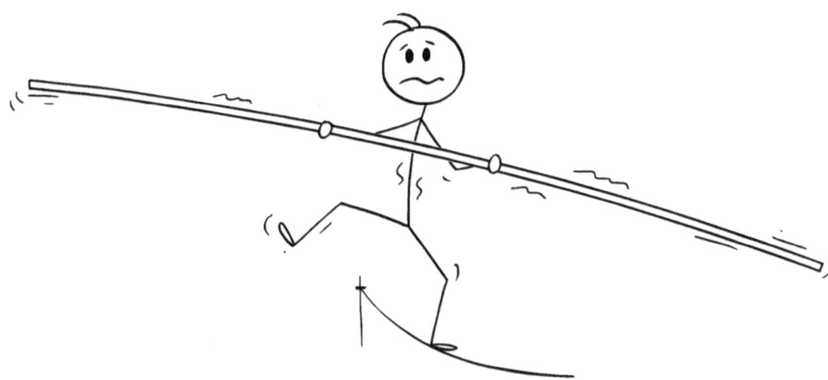

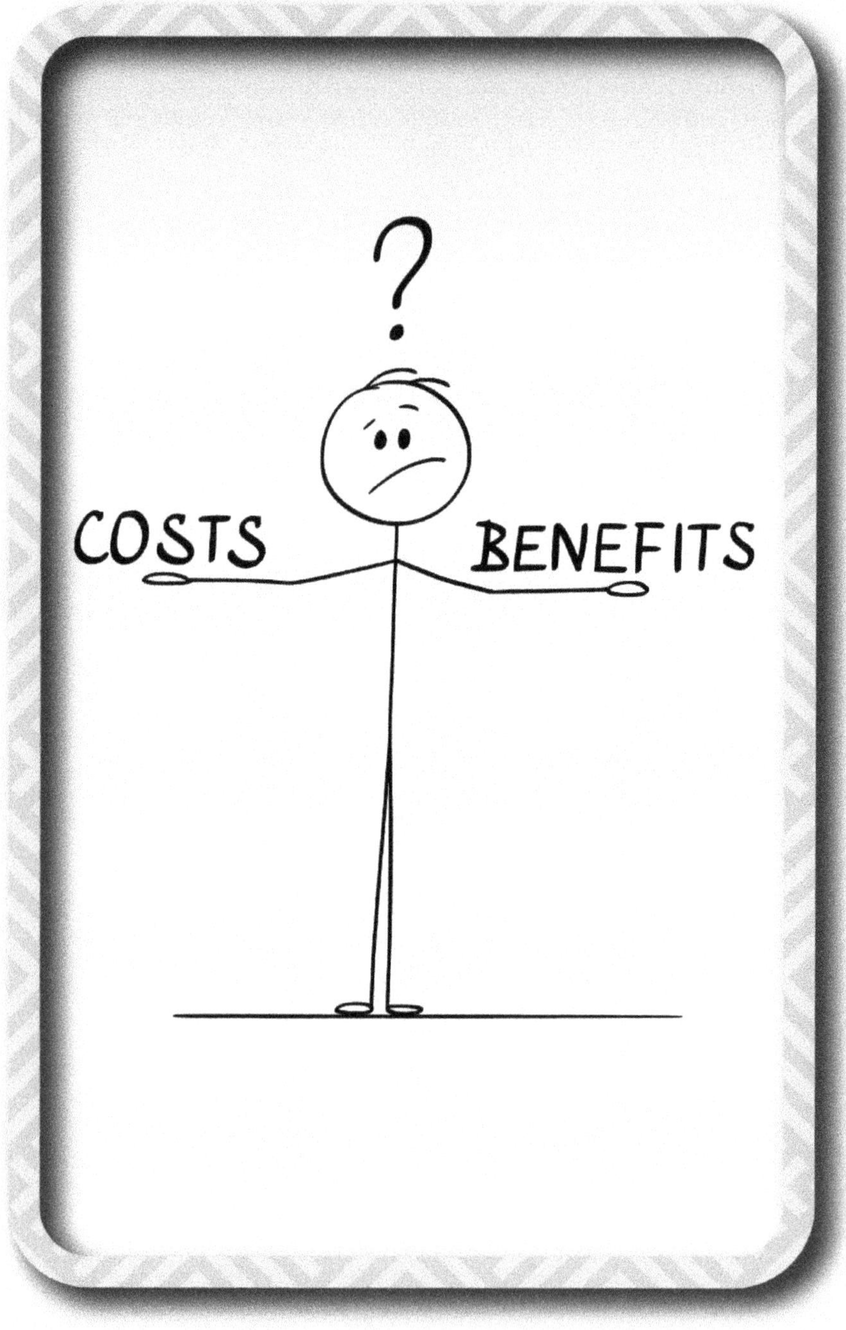
?
COSTS
BENEFITS

Sample List

Grey Area ⚑

Take a nap vs. Sleeping all day
A piece of chocolate vs. Pint of ice cream
Flirting vs. Promiscuous unsafe sex
Checking social media vs. Doom scrolling
One glass of wine vs. A bottle of wine
Window shopping vs. Excessive spending

Your Personal Grey Areas

Are there any grey area coping skills that you currently use or have used in the past?

____

____

____

____

6
Categories

Chapter 4 Six Category Overview

Six Categories of Coping Overview

Alright, it's finally time to dive into the good stuff! I've been hyping up these six coping skill categories, so get ready to organize your toolkit like a pro because here they come!

Each category represents a different approach to coping, allowing you to tailor your response to fit the situation. By organizing and listing positive coping skills into these six categories, you will optimize the effectiveness of your customized coping skill toolbox you are working to create.

It's important to note that there may be some overlap between the categories. For example, practicing yoga can provide both physical relief and serve as a mindfulness skill. That's perfectly okay! The goal is to have a diverse range of coping strategies at your disposal.

After we discuss each category, you'll find a sample page with a list of examples. But don't stop there! Take a moment to brainstorm your own ideas in each category. Then, flip to the back of the book where you'll find your blank "Your Personal Coping Skills Toolkit" template ready to be customized and filled out by you. Stuck on ideas? No worries! Just flip through the "Coping Skills Ideas" section for some inspiration. Here we go!

Drum roll please 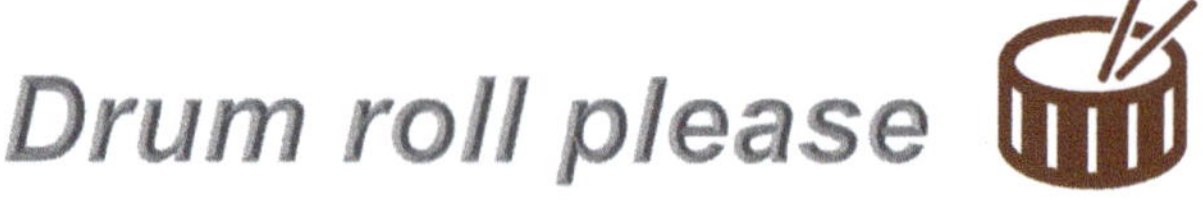

The 6 Categories

Without further ado, let's introduce the six categories:

1 **Process:** This category focuses on actively engaging with your thoughts and emotions. Process coping skills involve talking things out, whether it's with a trusted friend, therapist, or through journaling.

2 **Distract:** Distraction is not the same as avoidance. Distraction coping skills help shift your focus away from overwhelming thoughts or emotions, temporarily allowing you to take a step back and gain perspective.

3 **Self-soothe:** When you are in fight, flight or freeze, self-soothing coping skills come into play. These techniques utilize the five senses – sight, sound, touch, taste, and smell – which calm your central nervous system.

4 **Physical:** Physical coping skills involve actions that directly impact your body. These can include nutrition, progressive muscle relaxation, or engaging in activities that release tension and promote physical well-being.

5 **Positive Self-talk:** Your inner dialogue plays a powerful role in how you perceive and respond to the world. Positive self-talk coping skills involve cultivating a supportive, motivating and encouraging inner monologue and countering negative thoughts and beliefs.

6 **Mindfulness:** Being present in the here and now is a key component of mindfulness coping skills. These techniques help

you ground yourself in the present moment, fostering awareness, acceptance, and a sense of peace.

In the following chapters, we'll delve deeper into each category, providing a range of coping skills and strategies for you to explore. Remember, building your personal coping skill toolbox is a journey, so be patient with yourself as you discover what works best for you. Let's get started!

Chapter 5 Processing

CATEGORY 1: PROCESSING INFORMATION

Let's get right into the first category and the reason that therapists are so popular. Processing! In this chapter, we will explore the importance of processing information as well as brainstorm some coping skills that fit into this category. Your ability to effectively process information greatly influences how you respond to challenges and stressors in your life. By understanding how you process information and leveraging the knowledge to choose better coping skills, you can enhance your problem-solving abilities and reduce feelings of being overwhelmed.

Ways To Process

One of the most effective ways to seek support is by talking about our problems or journaling our thoughts and feelings. When we keep everything bottled up inside, it can feel overwhelming and isolating. However, when we share our burdens with someone else, whether it's a trusted friend, family member, or therapist, we allow ourselves to release some of the tension, gain insight and see things from a new perspective. When we talk out loud about our difficulties, we give ourselves the opportunity to hear our own thoughts and feelings. Sometimes, simply verbalizing our concerns can help us gain clarity and insight into the situation. It's like untangling a knot - as we speak, the jumbled thoughts in our mind start to unravel, and we begin to see things more clearly.

You will find that you naturally process different information with different people in your life. For instance, you might discuss work stress with a coworker and family issues with a sibling. Take a moment to think about the people in your life who help you process your thoughts and emotions. Is it a best friend, a cousin, or perhaps your mom? By sharing our burdens, we give others the chance to offer their insights, advice, or simply a listening ear. Sometimes, all we need is someone who can empathize and validate our feelings.

The more supports you have, the better... although if you feel like you lack supportive people, there are still plenty of options. Consider talking to a therapist, having a conversation with yourself out loud (maybe in the car!), join an online or in-person support group or express your thoughts and feelings through journaling.

Writing down our thoughts and emotions can have a similar effect to talking out loud. It allows us to externalize our internal struggles and also provides a safe space for self-reflection. As we put pen to paper, we can explore our emotions, fears, and hopes without judgment. It's a way to process our thoughts at our own pace and in our own words, giving us the freedom to express ourselves fully.

Part of processing emotion and stress for better mental health is recognizing you are struggling and asking for help as you need it. The level of support required will vary depending on the severity of the distress, ranging from discomfort to crisis situation. Sometimes you need help problem-solving, require help finding resources, need someone to volley ideas back and forth or you just want a sympathetic listener. However, if you believe that you pose a threat to yourself or others, it is imperative to immediately contact emergency services or visit the nearest hospital emergency room for immediate assistance.

How We Process Information

Our brains are remarkable organs that constantly process and interpret information from the world around us. When faced with a problem or stressful situation, different parts of our brain are engaged to help us make sense of what's happening and formulate a response.

Research has shown that when you verbalize your thoughts and feelings, such as by talking out loud, you engage areas of the brain involved in problem-solving and emotional regulation. This process allows you to gain clarity, organize your thoughts, and explore potential solutions more effectively than if you simply kept your thoughts internalized. When you ruminate on thoughts and do not process out loud or by writing, it can create worry, distorted thinking and amplify stress.

Your cognitive processes are deeply intertwined with your ability to communicate and express yourself. Verbalizing your thoughts not only engages the areas of your brain responsible for problem-solving and emotional regulation but also serves as a channel for understanding and connecting with others. In a way, your words act as bridges between the complexities of your inner world and the shared reality you inhabit with those around you. Profound, right?

Consider a scenario where someone has run into a challenging problem with a decision that is needed to be made at work. By discussing their thoughts and concerns with coworkers, they not only gain valuable insights but also stimulate cognitive processes that might have remained dormant otherwise. Through dialogue, they can explore different perspectives, weigh the pros and cons, and ultimately arrive at a more informed decision. This exchange not only enriches their own understanding but also fosters collaboration and mutual support within the team.

When you bottle up our thoughts and emotions, they can fester and grow unchecked, leading to increased stress and anxiety. Without an outlet for expression, your mind may distort and expand information contributing to consternation, replaying the same worries and fears on an endless loop. By vocalizing your concerns, you disrupt this cycle and create space for constructive problem-solving and emotional regulation. In doing so, you not only alleviate the burden on your mind but also pave the way for healthier, more resilient ways of coping with adversity.

Verbalizing your thoughts enhances the benefits gained through self-reflection and introspection. As you articulate your innermost thoughts and emotions, you are forced to confront them in a more tangible way. This process of externalization can offer new insights and revelations, leading to greater self-awareness and personal growth. In essence, the spoken word serves as a mirror, reflecting back the nuances of your own psyche and inviting you to engage with them more deeply. This is a primary objective of therapy!

The Supporting Research

Let's look at the science. Numerous studies have highlighted the efficacy of various processing techniques in improving cognitive functioning and emotional well-being. Here are some examples:

Research conducted by Professor Matthew Lieberman and his colleagues at the University of California, Los Angeles (UCLA), has demonstrated the benefits of verbalizing thoughts and feelings. Their studies using functional magnetic resonance imaging (fMRI) have shown increased activity in brain regions associated with problem-solving and emotional regulation when individuals speak about their experiences (Lieberman, 2019).

Studies in psychotherapy research have consistently shown the effectiveness of therapeutic dialogue in promoting emotional processing and symptom reduction. Meta-analyses have found that various forms of talk therapy, including cognitive-behavioral therapy (CBT) and psychodynamic therapy, lead to significant improvements in psychological well-being (Cuijpers et al., 2016).

Research on social support has consistently demonstrated its importance in coping with stress and adversity. Studies have shown that individuals who receive support from friends and family members report lower levels of psychological distress and better overall mental health (Thoits, 2011).

Studies examining the therapeutic benefits of journaling have found that writing about emotional experiences can lead to improvements in mood, stress reduction, and increased self-awareness. Expressive writing has been associated with enhanced emotional processing and greater psychological resilience (Baikie & Wilhelm, 2005).

The research cited above explains the importance of this category. When facing a difficult dilemma or stressful situation, consider reaching out for support and process your stress and emotion to help resolve or cope with the distress. It's important to remember that seeking support is not a sign of weakness, but rather a sign of strength. It takes courage to acknowledge our struggles and ask for help. By doing so, we give ourselves the opportunity to find solutions, gain new perspectives, and ultimately cope with the challenges life throws our way. Talking out loud or journaling are going to have a greater benefit than simply thinking things over in your mind.

Building Your Toolkit

Now that you have a better understanding of the first category, check out the sample list at the end of this chapter and jot down ideas of how you can process information and identify your supportive people. Then, before moving on to the next chapter, flip to the back of the book and copy what you have written in the corresponding category on the "Your Personal Coping Skills Toolkit." Remember, having only a couple of ideas is okay. Begin with a few and gradually add more to your list over time. You can check out the bonus section at the end of the book for inspiration.

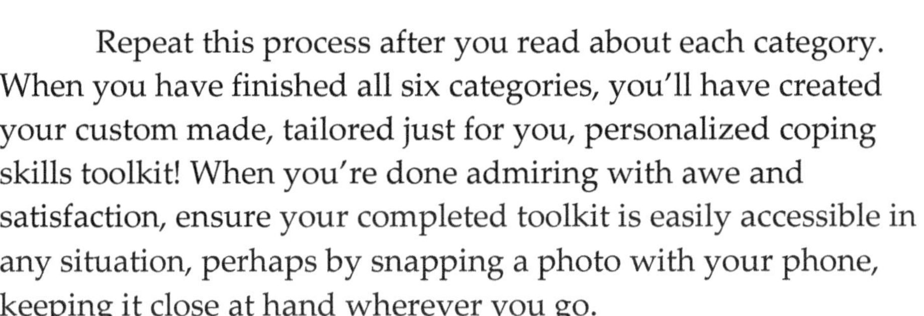

Repeat this process after you read about each category. When you have finished all six categories, you'll have created your custom made, tailored just for you, personalized coping skills toolkit! When you're done admiring with awe and satisfaction, ensure your completed toolkit is easily accessible in any situation, perhaps by snapping a photo with your phone, keeping it close at hand wherever you go.

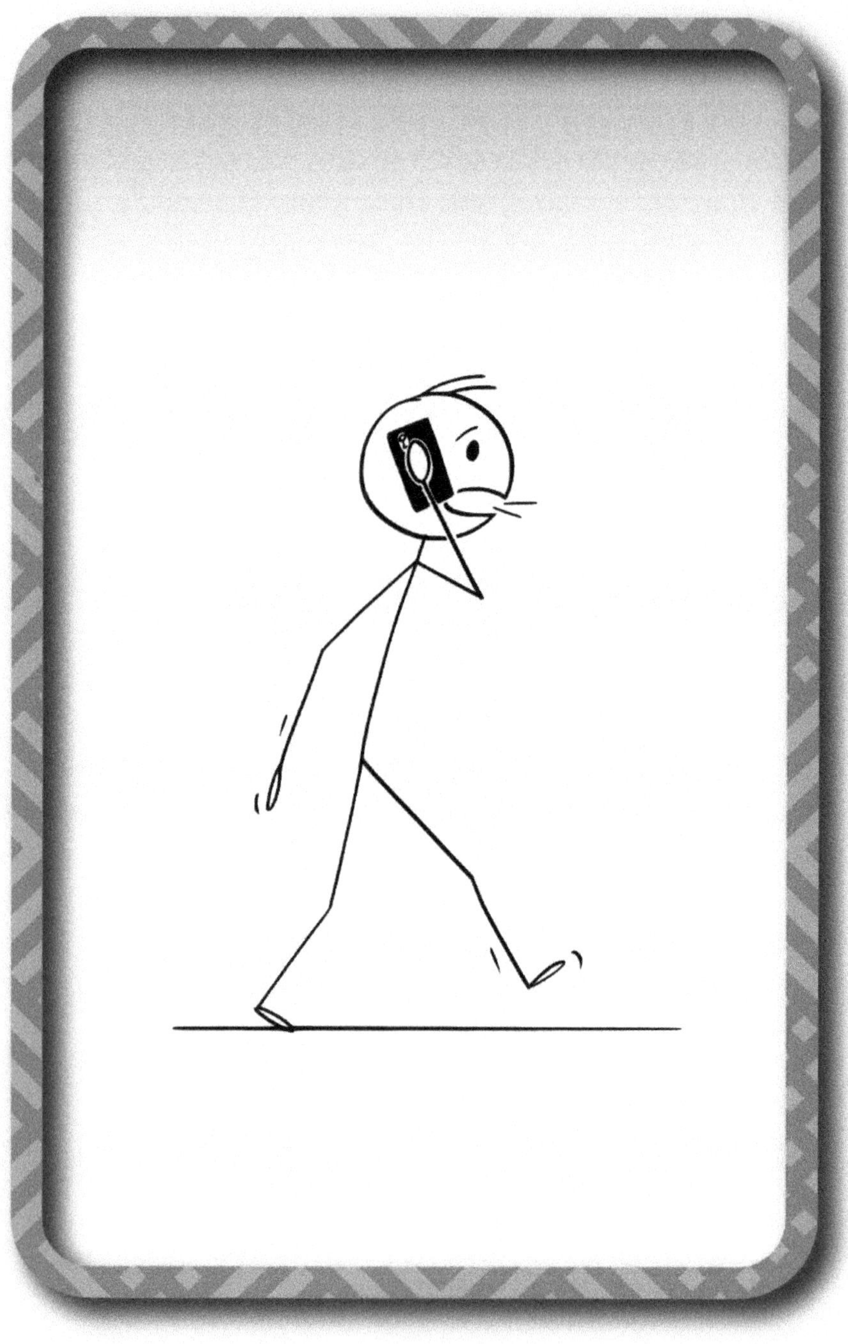

Sample List

Process

Get support from a therapist

Talk to your mom

Text your best friend

Tell your cat

Create a gratitude journal

Write a song about it

Jot down some ideas of your own

____

____

____

____

____

Now flip to the back and write these ideas in the corresponding section in "Your Personal Coping Skill Toolkit."

Chapter 6 Distracting

CATEGORY 2: DISTRACTION TECHNIQUES

This section explores the second category on our list, distraction techniques. Distracting can be incredibly helpful in managing overwhelming thoughts and emotions. Distraction techniques are all about shifting your focus away from what's currently causing you distress. They can give you the breathing room to come back with a fresh perspective. When you give your brain a break from the stressors, you create space for new ideas and solutions to bubble up to the surface.

Distinguishing Distraction from Avoidance

Now, it's important to note that distraction isn't the same as avoidance and it is important to draw a clear distinction between the two. While distraction and avoidance may appear similar on the surface, they differ in their underlying intentions and outcomes. Distraction coping skills allow you to take a momentary step back, giving yourself a breather without ignoring the problem altogether. Think of distraction as hitting the pause button. Avoidance however, involves completely ignoring or denying the issue at hand by pretending the problem does not exist or attempting not to experience the negative emotions.

Not to distract from the topic, (ha, dad joke,) let's take a moment to explore avoidance a little further before discussing how distracting techniques can help. Avoidance can seem like a tempting escape hatch when faced with challenging emotions or situations. But there's a catch: avoidance only offers temporary relief and in the long run it doesn't address the root cause and can even make things worse.

Sometimes we inadvertently suppress our emotions or develop coping mechanisms that serve to avoid. One example is dissociation, where individuals mentally detach from their surroundings or emotions as a defense mechanism. It's like watching life through a foggy lens, where everything feels distant and unreal. Another related phenomenon is depersonalization, where individuals feel disconnected from themselves, almost as if they're watching their own life unfold from the sidelines.

Some other examples of avoidance are isolating, social withdrawal, passive communication, procrastination and substance use. The more you use avoidance either unintentionally or as a choice to dodge uncomfortable feelings or situations, the bigger the problem can grow like a cancer festering beneath the surface. It's like trying to hold a beach ball underwater—the harder you push it down, the more forcefully it pops back up. Avoidance takes a lot of mental resources and expending that emotional energy to avoid can hinder quality of life and personal growth.

Instead of resorting to avoidance, it is necessary to face emotions head-on. That doesn't mean you have to tackle everything at once—it's about taking small steps towards acceptance and understanding. Meanwhile, if the emotions are too intense or the issue becomes overwhelming, that is when distraction techniques can become valuable tools to give a necessary and temporary reprieve.

Why Distracting Helps

Here's how distraction coping skills can be beneficial:

Provide Temporary Relief: If thoughts or feelings are overwhelming, distracting can provide temporary relief. By engaging in an activity that captures your attention, you can get a break from the intensity of your feelings.

Shift in Focus: When you're consumed by negative thoughts or emotions, it's easy to lose sight of anything else. Distraction techniques help shift focus onto something else, even if just for a little while. This shift can break the cycle of rumination and give your mind a chance to reset.

Calming Effect: Certain distraction activities, such as listening to music, or taking a nap can have a calming effect on your mind and body.

Gain Perspective: Stepping away from a stressful situation through distraction can provide a fresh perspective when you return to it. Sometimes, taking a break allows you to see things more clearly or come up with new solutions to challenges.

Now, let's explore some distraction techniques that you can incorporate into your coping toolbox:

ENTERTAINMENT: Escapism is a valid form of distracting. Forms of entertainment such as reading, scrolling on the phone, watching TV or movies or playing games help transport your mind to a different place.

HOBBIES: Whether it's painting, knitting, gardening, or playing a musical instrument, immersing yourself in a hobby can be a great way to distract from stressors.

ENJOYING NATURE: Spending time outdoors, whether it's taking a hike in the woods or simply sitting in a park, can help you disconnect from stressors and focus on the external world instead of internal turmoil.

In therapy, when asked, "What coping skills do you currently use?" many people often list distraction techniques. Distracting is a completely legitimate form of positive coping, so don't hesitate to experiment with different distraction activities and find what works best for you. However, coping through distraction may not always be the only coping skill category to explore. While distracting can provide relief in the moment, it's essential to address underlying issues and develop long-term coping strategies as well. Remember, distraction techniques are just one of the six categories in our coping toolkit so let's explore our remaining categories!

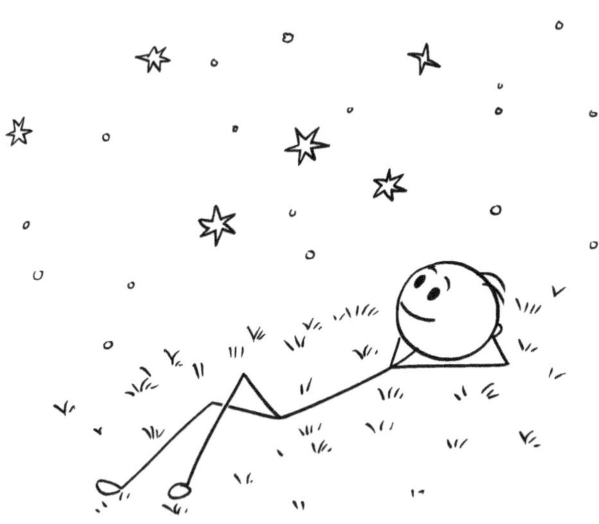

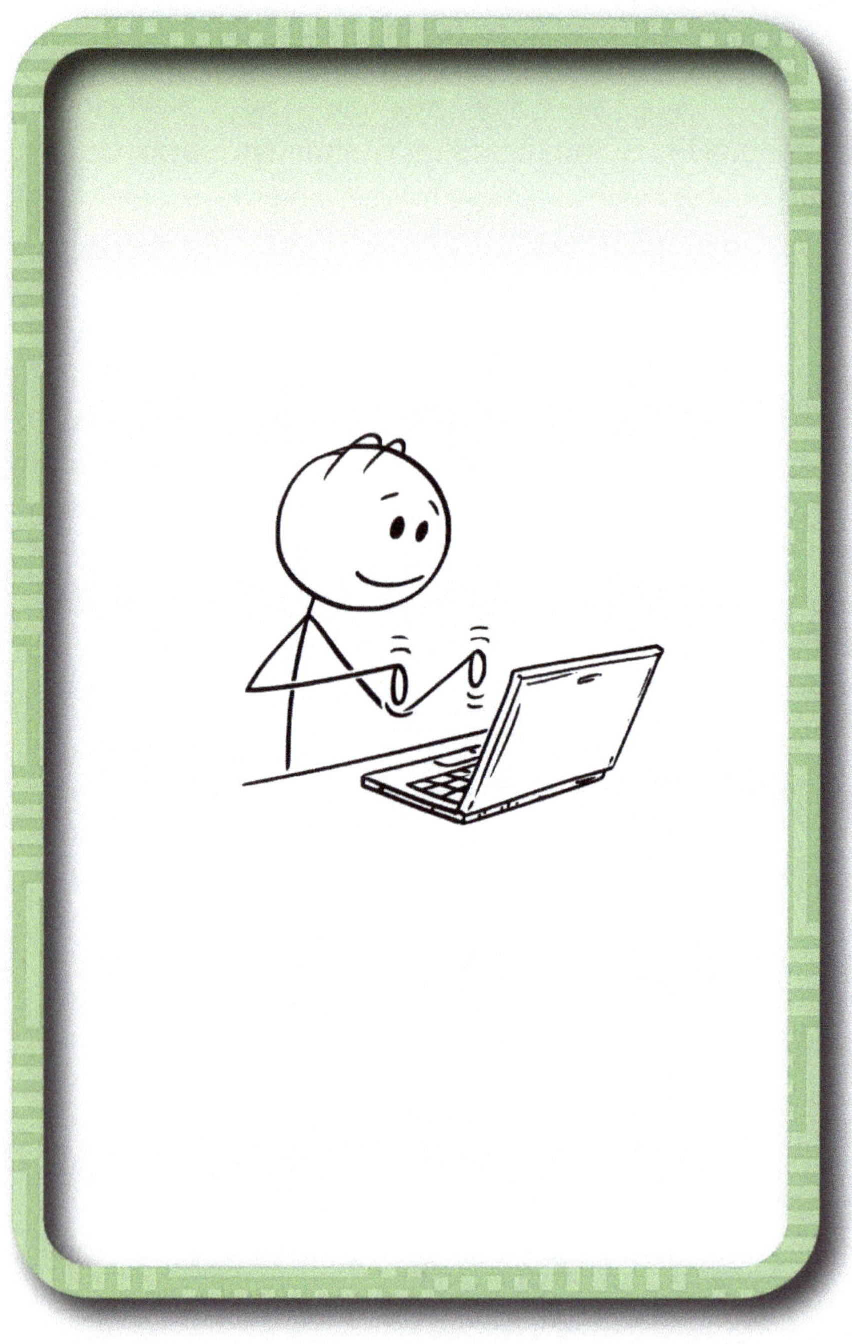

Sample List

Distract

Catch up on laundry

Watch TV

Go see a movie

Read a book

Play a video game

Learn the glockenspiel

Jot down some ideas of your own

____

____

____

____

____

Chapter 7 Self-Soothe

CATEGORY 3: SELF SOOTHE

Welcome to the third category! In this chapter, we'll explore self-soothing techniques, which are invaluable tools for managing stress and overwhelming emotions. Self-soothing techniques are particularly effective because they engage your senses, helping to regulate your autonomic nervous system and bring about a sense of calm.

As children, we naturally possess instinctive habits of self-soothing, such as thumb-sucking, rocking, and cuddling blankets. As adults, we also have the opportunity to explore and utilize an array of self-soothing methods to ease stress.

Autonomic Nervous System (ANS)

Before we dive into specific techniques, let's briefly understand the autonomic nervous system. The ANS is responsible for the regulation of involuntary bodily processes such as digestion, heart rate, blood pressure and respiration. It is comprised of two main branches: the sympathetic nervous system (SNS) and the parasympathetic nervous system (PNS).

Sympathetic Nervous System (SNS)

The sympathetic nervous system is the branch of the ANS associated with the body's "fight, flight or freeze" response. When you encounter a perceived threat or stressor, the SNS is activated, leading to increased heart rate, rapid breathing, and heightened alertness.

FLIGHT, FIGHT, FREEZE: In times of perceived danger or threat, the body's natural survival mechanism naturally kicks into gear, leading to what is commonly known as "fight, flight, or freeze." This response prepares your body for strenuous physical activity that may be needed in order to respond to the threat and survive.

You can think of it as your body's survival mode. Imagine you're walking in the woods, minding your own business, when suddenly, you spot a huge bear charging at you! Your heart starts pounding, your breath quickens, and your muscles tense up. This is your SNS kicking into high gear, getting you ready to either fight that bear or run like the wind to escape. It's a warning system that tells your body, "Emergency! Act now!" It's all about gearing up your body for action in response to stress or danger.

FIGHT: This response might prepare you to fight back, mobilizing energy and increasing alertness to confront the bear head-on.

FLIGHT: Maybe your body senses that the bear will win, therefore prepares to flee, seek safety and escape.

FREEZE: In some situations, your body may enter a state of immobility or "freeze," which hopefully will communicate to the bear that you are boring and not a threat.

While the fight, flight, freeze response is essential for survival, like when encountering a bear, it can become maladaptive when activated in common daily non-life-threatening situations such as relationship issues or job pressure, leading to chronic stress, anxiety, and other health problems.

Parasympathetic Nervous System (PNS)

In contrast, the parasympathetic nervous system promotes a state of relaxation and restoration. Known as your "rest and digest" state, when activated, slows your heart rate, improves digestion, and promotes feelings of calmness and relaxation. When you are calm and relaxed you are better able to problem solve. You can use the distress thermometer discussed in chapter 2 to assess your current stress level. If you are a lower number such as 1, 2 or 3, the PNS is likely in control.

Vagus Nerve

The vagus nerve is the body's built-in mechanism. As the heart of the ANS, the vagus nerve is a cranial nerve that is a major player in regulating your body's stress response. The vagus nerve travels from the brainstem to various organs throughout your entire body effecting many body functions including heart rate, immune system, digestion and breathing rate.

The vagus nerve acts as a switch between the SNS and PNS, helping to maintain balance and homeostasis in the body. When the switch is activated, it stimulates the PNS, promoting relaxation and quieting the stress response. Techniques that activate the vagus nerve in order to stimulate the PNS can be particularly effective in reducing anxiety and promoting emotional well-being.

Vagal Tone

Vagal tone refers to the activity level of the vagus nerve. Essentially, individuals with high vagal tone are better equipped to cope with stressors, as their bodies can more efficiently return to a state of calm after a stressful event. Poor vagal tone may manifest as heightened stress levels, difficulty managing emotions, and increased susceptibility to health issues like digestive problems or cardiovascular issues.

There are several ways to enhance vagal tone, including relaxation, stress reduction exercises, and physical activity. By improving vagal tone, you may experience reduced anxiety, better digestion, and even enhanced immune function. Thankfully, even small changes in lifestyle habits can make a big difference in nurturing and maintaining healthy vagal tone for a more balanced and vibrant life.

Using The 5 Senses

Self-soothing techniques that engage the five senses can be incredibly effective in calming the central nervous system and promoting relaxation. As you explore self-soothing techniques, in addition to stimulating the vagus nerve, consider incorporating sensory memories. We can use our senses to elicit happy or calming memories. Our senses are closely linked to memory, and certain smells, sounds, tastes, and sights can evoke powerful emotions and memories from the past. By intentionally incorporating sensory experiences associated with positive or calming memories, we can enhance the effectiveness of self-soothing techniques and promote emotional health.

Now, let's explore how your five senses can help to soothe the autonomic nervous system, leverage sensory memories and promote relaxation. We'll look at each sense—sight, sound, smell, taste, and touch—and discuss specific techniques you can incorporate into your daily routine.

SIGHT: What we see can have a profound impact on our emotions and state of mind. Plus, visual stimuli have a strong impact on memory recall. Reflect on images or scenes that bring you joy or peace. It could be a photo of a loved one, a beautiful landscape, or artwork that holds special meaning for you. Surround yourself with these visual reminders to evoke positive emotions and soothe your mind. Engaging in activities that bring you joy and peace, such as watching a sunset, flipping through a photo album of cherished memories, or simply observing nature, can help calm the mind and reduce stress.

SOUND: What we hear has the ability to influence our mood and physiology. Sound is another powerful trigger for memory and emotion. Consider creating a playlist of songs that uplift your spirits or remind you of happy times. Listening to familiar tunes can transport you back to cherished memories and provide comfort during times of stress or anxiety. Listening to a soothing voice, nature sounds, or white noise can help quiet the mind and promote relaxation. Experiment with different types of auditory stimuli to find what works best for you.

SMELL: Aromatherapy, the use of scents to promote healing and well-being, can be a powerful tool for self-soothing. The sense of smell is processed by the limbic system which is the part of your brain responsible for your memory and emotions.

Certain scents can instantly transport us to different times and places. Experiment with using scents that evoke positive memories, such as the aroma of freshly baked cookies, the scent of a favorite flower, or the smell of a comforting meal cooking in the kitchen. Essential oils such as lavender, chamomile, and peppermint have been shown to have calming effects on the nervous system. Some people use a diffuser or inhale essential oils directly to experience their benefits.

TASTE: What we taste can be used in various ways to self-soothe, however, don't forget to pay attention to the grey area that we discussed earlier. Having food in your belly can activate the PNS. Taste memories are deeply ingrained in our minds and can evoke strong emotional responses. Indulge in foods or beverages that remind you of happy times or special occasions. Comforting beverages such as a cup of hot chocolate can be soothing, although watch out for caffeine beverages which can increase anxiety. Whether it's a warm cup of chai tea, a piece of chocolate, or a homemade meal prepared with love, savoring these tastes can bring comfort and relaxation.

TOUCH: Physical touch has been shown to release oxytocin, a feel-good hormone that contributes to feelings of bonding and relaxation. Physical sensations can also trigger memories and emotions. Surround yourself with textures that bring you comfort, such as a soft blanket, cozy sweater, or smooth stone. Engage in activities that involve tactile stimulation, such as gardening, crafting, or simply running your fingers through sand or playing with slime. Engaging in gentle self-massage, hugging a loved one, or simply petting a furry friend can be a very effective way to self-soothe.

In this chapter, we've explored the power of self-soothing techniques in managing stress and promoting emotional well-being. By engaging your senses, using the power of sensory memories and stimulating the vagus nerve, you can effectively regulate your autonomic nervous system and more quickly return to a sense of calm and relaxation after stress.

Remember, self-soothing is a type of skill that works to varying degrees depending on the situation. Experiment with different kinds of self-soothing and find what works best for you. Before you know it, you will effortlessly and automatically reach for these effective coping skills to help you deescalate and navigate through life's challenges.

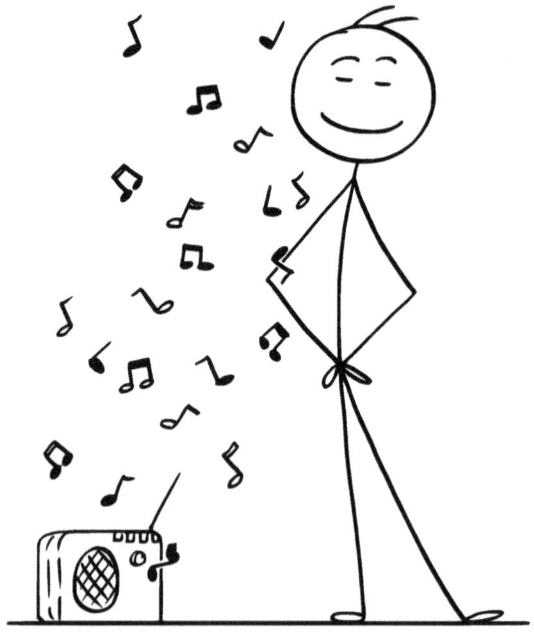

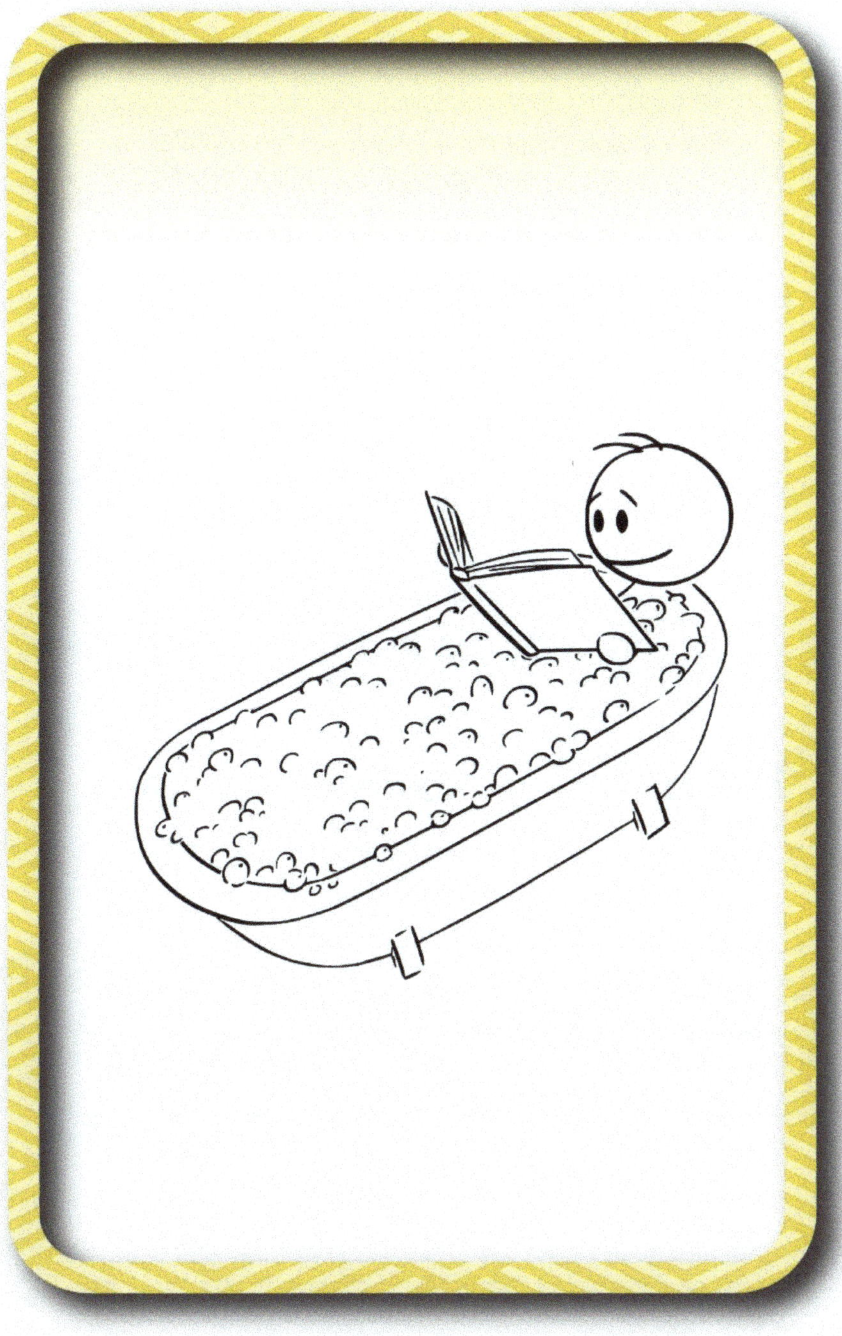

Sample List

Self-Soothe

Pet your dog

Put on cozy pajamas

Drink herbal tea

Watch nature in your yard

Take a bubble bath

Light a lavender candle

Jot down some ideas of your own

____

____

____

____

____

Chapter 8 Physical

The next category is all about physical and somatic coping skills. These techniques focus on the body's response to stress and can be incredibly effective in managing difficult emotions and situations.

Rule Out Medical Causes

When struggling with ongoing stress or emotional disturbance, it is crucial to rule out any potential medical conditions that could be mistaken for mental health concerns. Physical health and mental well-being are closely intertwined and symptoms can sometimes mirror each other. It is important to make sure stress and mood disturbance do not stem directly from an underlying medical problem.

Seeing medical providers for regular visits as recommended can be a game-changer in catching any health-related issues early on. Routine checkups provide an opportunity to keep tabs on your overall health, spotting any issues and tackling concerns before they spiral out of control. A proactive approach not only promotes physical health but also contributes to mental wellness by ensuring that any potential medical causes are promptly identified and treated.

Allowing collaboration between providers, whether it's a therapist, psychiatrist, primary care physician or chiropractor can offer comprehensive care with everyone on the same page. You know, mental health and physical health are like two peas in a pod - they coexist and aren't mutually exclusive, meaning what's going on in your mind can have a big impact on your body, and vice versa!

The Bodies Response to Stress

Before we dive into specific coping techniques, let's take a moment to understand how stress affects the body. As we touched on in the previous chapter, when we experience stress, whether it's from work, relationships, or other sources, our bodies go into a state of heightened alertness often referred to as the "fight, flight or freeze" response. When this occurs, we experience a physiological response. For example, our heart rate increases, muscles tense up, and adrenaline surges through our system.

While this response can be helpful in short bursts, chronic stress can take a toll on our physical and mental health. It can lead to a range of symptoms, including muscle tension, headaches, digestive issues, and even weakened immune function. Additionally, stress can become stored in the body, manifesting as tightness or discomfort in certain areas.

Sleep, Water and Nutrition

In my therapy practice, I am constantly assessing sleep, water intake and nutrition. Inadequate amounts of these seemingly obvious human needs can sometimes be an underlying source or contributing factor in our ability or inability to effectively cope. Ironically, mental health issues themselves can disrupt our sleep, hydration, and dietary routines, creating a harmful cycle. So, before we use and explore other coping techniques, it's essential to optimize and understand the impact of sleep, water, and nutrition in managing stress. These basic needs are often overlooked but play a crucial role in supporting our mental health.

SLEEP: Sleep supports memory consolidation, boosts cognitive function, enhances mood, promotes physical rejuvenation, and strengthens the immune system. Research has shown that chronic sleep deprivation can contribute to increased stress levels, impaired cognitive function, and mood disturbances. Getting quality sleep each night will support your body's ability to cope and heal. If you struggle with sleep, consider seeing a sleep specialist. Set up a bedtime routine that incorporates relaxation techniques to help your body anticipate sleep.

Have you ever heard of the term circadian rhythm? Your circadian rhythm is your body's natural 24-hour clock that regulates your body functions such as hormone release, body temperature, when to wake, get tired, feel hungry and have the urge to use the bathroom. Your body loves predictability and routine. When you have an erratic schedule, the body does not know when to secrete natural chemicals such a melatonin to make us sleepy.

WATER: Staying hydrated is key to maintaining optimal bodily function, including the regulation of stress hormones. Dehydration can exacerbate feelings of fatigue and tension, making it harder to cope with stress. In fact, look up all the benefits of water… Go ahead, I'll wait. That probably took a while because water has so many benefits. Adequate water intake is essential for feeling well and helping our body function. Therefore, make sure you are drinking enough water and be mindful of increasing your intake during times of heightened stress or physical activity.

NUTRITION: Maintaining a nutritious, healthy and well-balanced diet is crucial for effectively managing stress. Certain foods, such as those high in sugar and processed ingredients, can actually increase feelings of stress and anxiety. Focus on nourishing your body with wholesome foods that support overall health.

Your body relies on minerals and vitamins to carry out body functions. As you would not expect your car to go without fuel, you cannot reasonably expect your body to perform very well without adequate nutrition. It is equally important to avoid foods that can have a negative impact. It may be wise to limit caffeine on days that you are experiencing anxiety.

Somatic Coping Skills

Now that we've covered the basics, let's explore some specific physical coping techniques that focus on the body's response to stress.

BREATHING EXERCISES: Controlled breathing is a simple yet effective way to deescalate. It can activate the parasympathetic response, effectively calming the nervous system. There are many types of breathing techniques. Try practicing diaphragmatic breathing by inhaling deeply through your nose, allowing your abdomen to expand, and exhale slowly through your mouth like you are blowing out a candle.

PROGRESSIVE MUSCLE RELAXATION (PMR): PMR involves tensing and relaxing muscles in the body one at a time in order to relieve stress. This technique can help release physical tension and promote relaxation. Start by tensing your muscles tightly for a few seconds, then slowly releasing and allowing them to relax completely. Move through each muscle group, from your head to your toes, paying attention to any areas of tension or discomfort.

MINDFUL MOVEMENT: Engaging in gentle movement practices such as yoga, tai chi, or even basic stretching can help release tension and promote relaxation. These practices encourage mindful awareness of the body and breath, fostering a sense of groundedness and peace. Research has shown that regular practice of mindful movement can reduce stress hormones and improve overall mental health.

MASSAGE THERAPY: Massage therapy is a hands-on approach to relieving muscle tension and promoting relaxation. Research has shown that massage can reduce levels of the stress hormone cortisol while increasing levels of neurotransmitters associated with relaxation, such as serotonin and dopamine. Whether you get a massage at a fancy day spa or simply self-massage at home, incorporating massage into your routine can be a valuable tool for coping with stress.

PHYSICAL ACTIVITY: Regular physical activity is a go-to for improving both physical and mental health. Exercise triggers the release of endorphins, which are hormones that act as natural pain-relievers and mood boosters. Experts recommend at least 30 minutes of moderate exercise most days of the week, whether it's going for a walk, jogging, swimming, or participating in your favorite sport.

BODY SCAN / BIOFEEDBACK: **A** body scan is a type of meditation that brings awareness to different parts of the body, allowing you to notice any sensations, discomfort, or areas of tension. Biofeedback, on the other hand, refers to the body's innate ability to provide feedback about its internal state. For example, feeling your heart race in response to stress or sweating when you're nervous are forms of biofeedback. Essentially, biofeedback is your body's way of communicating with you, helping you become more aware of what's going on inside so you can respond accordingly.

Incorporating physical coping skills into your daily routine can provide powerful tools for managing stress and promoting overall well-being. By prioritizing sleep, water, and nutrition, along with routine checkups and practicing techniques such as breathing exercises, progressive muscle relaxation, and mindful movement, you can cultivate greater resilience in the face of life's challenges.

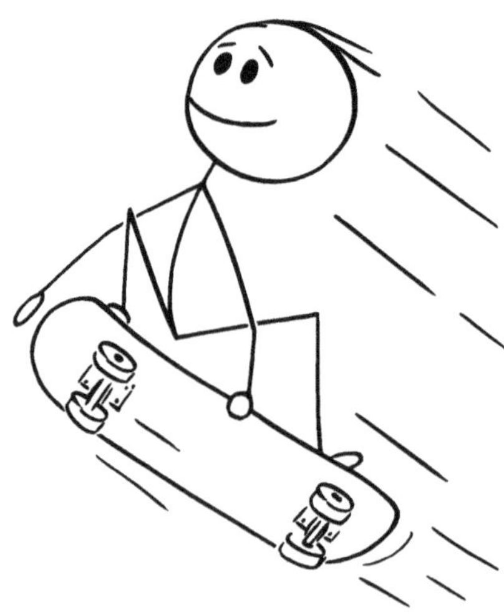

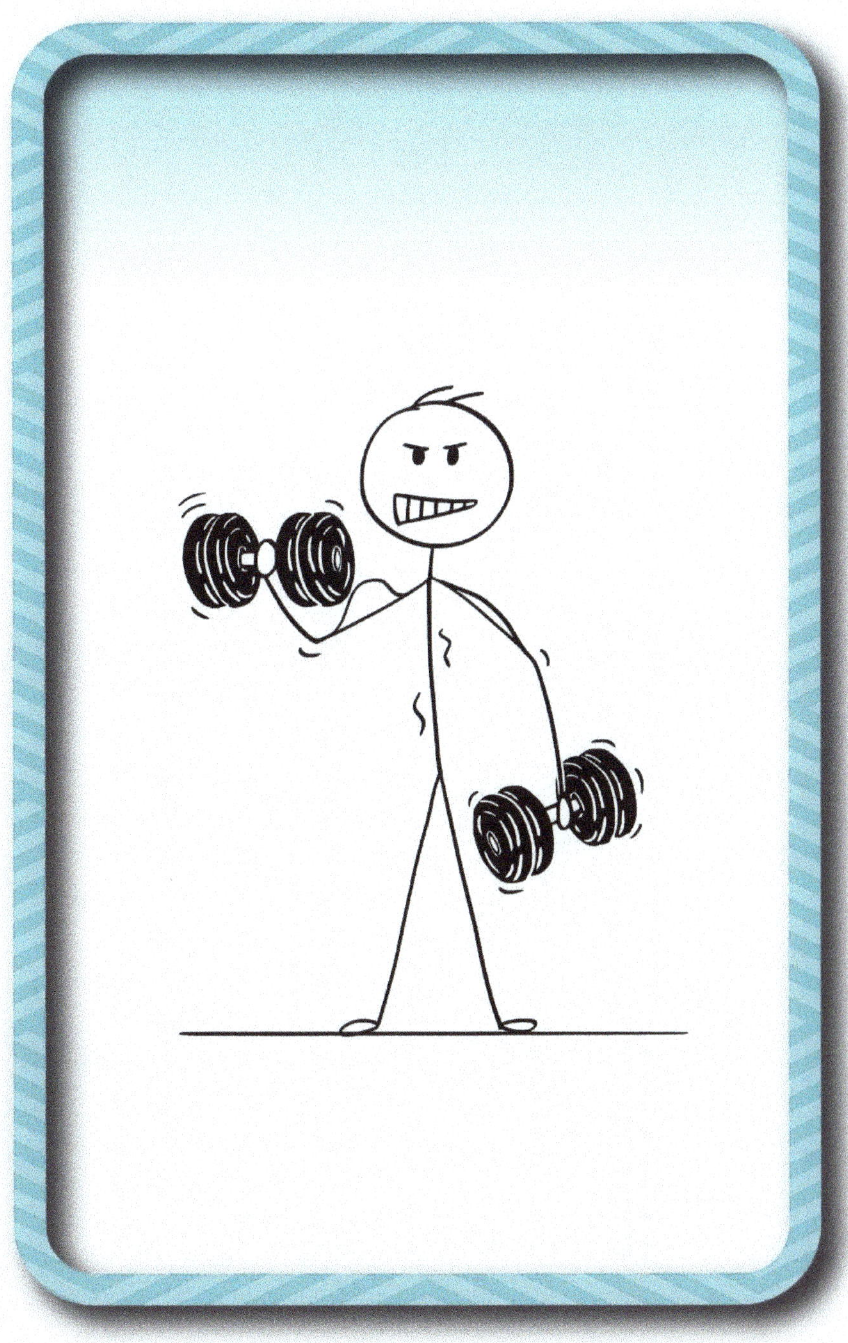

Sample List

Physical

Increase your sleep

See your doctor

Go to Pilates class

Get a massage

Do morning stretches

Ride your bike

Jot down some ideas of your own

____

____

____

____

Chapter 9 Positive Self-Talk

CATEGORY 5: POSITIVE SELF-TALK

In this chapter, we will explore the transformative effects of positive self-talk. But what is positive self-talk? It is your internal monologue. Think of it as your mental coach or the hype-man in your mind. It's you as your own personal cheerleader motivating and encouraging yourself from within.

How you think profoundly impacts your feelings, beliefs and behaviors. If you are generally a positive thinker, you are likely to take more opportunity risks, have increased confidence and greater cognitive resilience. In fact, being a positive thinker can lead to many benefits from having better interpersonal relationships to a higher quality of life overall.

Understanding Self-Talk

Have you ever thought about whether you are an optimist or a pessimist? Most people tend to lean positive or negative with their internal monologue and overall perceptions. My favorite analogy involves a famous depressed Disney donkey and his manic tiger friend. Let's say it was raining where they hang out in the woods. The pessimistic donkey may say, "What a miserable, wet and cold day." "Best that I should stay inside." The optimistic tiger might say, "Yay, how fun, it's raining!" "I can go out, splash in puddles and watch for rainbows!"

In this example, the stimulus "rain" was the same, however, how each thought about the rain changed, significantly impacting mood, feelings and behavior. By working to reframe your thoughts, you can reconceptualize a problem by seeing it from a different perspective.

Positive self-talk involves consciously choosing to be optimistic and encouraging with your thoughts. It's about challenging negative or self-defeating thoughts and replacing them with affirming and empowering ones. Doing this is crucial because how you think profoundly impacts your self-concept, your mood and how you interact with the world. Repetition and consistency are key factors in establishing neural pathways in the brain, making both positive and negative thinking more automatic and effortless over time. Really let that sink in for a moment. If you are continuously cranky and negative, that could become a neurocognitive predisposition! Everything from how you carry yourself and the choices you make to the risks you do or do not take will be impacted by how positively or negatively you perceive and manage internal and external stimuli.

Using Evidence-Based Methods

Using Cognitive Behavioral Therapy (CBT), Rational Emotive Behavior Therapy (REBT) or other evidenced based methods such as Acceptance & Commitment Therapy (ACT), can help you to restructure neuropathways in your brain. That's right! - These proven techniques are a way to literally remap your brain so that being a positive thinker becomes effortless and your default way of thinking.

Cognitive Behavioral Therapy (CBT)

As a widely recognized and extensively researched form of therapy, CBT focuses on the relationship between thoughts, feelings, and behaviors. According to CBT, your thoughts have a powerful impact on your feelings and behaviors. In other words, what you think directly influences how you feel and how you act. So, by changing your thoughts, you can change how you feel and how you respond to situations, ultimately leading to positive changes in your life.

CBT is not simply about gaslighting yourself into thinking happy thoughts. It involves a cognitive restructuring process that begins with gaining insight into recurring intrusive negative thoughts and their frequency. It also entails identifying cognitive distortions and correcting errors in thinking by challenging and replacing maladaptive thoughts with more positive and realistic ones. Through CBT, new neural pathways are created in the brain, promoting healthier thought patterns and behaviors over time.

Acceptance Commitment Therapy (ACT)

ACT helps you deal with life's challenges by accepting what you can't change and focusing on what truly matters to you. ACT teaches you to acknowledge feelings without getting tangled up in them. Instead of trying to push away painful emotions or pretend they don't exist, ACT encourages you to embrace them with compassion. It's about saying, "Hey, I'm feeling uncomfortable right now, and that's okay." ACT also involves taking actions in line with your core values, even when things get tough. It invites you to identify and explore the values and principles that give your life purpose and meaning.

Rational Emotive Behavior Therapy (REBT)

REBT is another evidence-based cognitive therapy that emphasizes the role of irrational beliefs in shaping emotional responses. According to REBT, it's not the events themselves that cause our emotional distress but rather our interpretations of those events. REBT teaches individuals to identify and dispute irrational beliefs, replacing them with more rational and constructive beliefs. Through this process, individuals can reduce their emotional disturbances and develop greater ability for emotional regulation.

The A-B-C-D-E method is a mnemonic device that summarizes this theory.

A – Activating event: Trigger such as an internal event (thought, physical symptom) or external event (observation, experience, situation.)

B – Belief: The resulting belief about the event and can sometimes be irrational.

C – Consequence: The behavior or negative thoughts or feelings that come from the belief.

D – Dispute: Using evidence to challenge an irrational belief.

E – Effect: The outcome of disputing the event.

Research studies have shown that evidence-based therapies such as CBT, ACT and REBT are effective in reducing or even eliminating health symptoms from issues such as depression and anxiety. By challenging irrational beliefs and adopting a more rational perspective, individuals can experience significant improvements in their mental health. There are many other evidence-based practices proven to help such as Behavioral Activation that we did not cover today. Isn't science fascinating?

Other Self-Talk Techniques

Now that we understand the theoretical foundations of positive self-talk, let's explore some other practical ways to implement this powerful coping skill into daily life.

INTERNAL VALIDATION: This form of positive self-talk involves acknowledging and affirming your own worth and value, independent of external validation or approval. Instead of seeking validation from others, you learn to trust and affirm yourself, recognizing your inherent worthiness as a human being.

Sometimes we tend to acknowledge the heckler in our mind and it is important to drown out or challenge that voice with an internal hype-man. The voice of that hype-man can be your own voice, your mother, your best friend or your favorite actor. Hey, it can be a crowd of cheerleaders or the voice of famous narrator James Earl Jones.

MANTRA: Used to empower, motivate or calm, these short positive words or statements are repeated to yourself in order to elicit the desired effect. They can serve as powerful reminders of your strengths, values, and goals. The world of marketing has leveraged the power of using mantras to drive consumerism and luckily you also can harness the power to improve your mental health.

A mantra can be a meaningful quote to inspire, a phrase that conveys an uplifting message, or a powerful word to meditate on to get you through a difficult moment. A mantra can be a very useful and multipurpose tool in your coping skill toolkit.

AFFIRMATIONS: An affirmation is a positive statement about yourself that can include positive traits related to your skills, appearance, personality, and assets. The word "affirmations" can sometimes produce an eye roll, and unfortunately, this therapeutic tool has become a go-to word for self-help satire (thanks, SNL However, this tried-and-true coping technique truly works to improve and reinforce a healthy self-concept. By repeating affirmations, you can enhance your self-confidence, self-esteem, and overall mental well-being.

They can be also powerful tools for self-improvement and personal growth. By helping you to focus on your positive traits and abilities, you can cultivate a positive mindset and manifest the reality you desire. Embracing affirmations as a regular practice can create a profound shift in your inner and outer worlds, leading to a more joyful existence. So, call them whatever you'd like… but use them as a helpful coping skill to improve your mental state.

GRATITUDE: A familiar concept to many, gratitude is the practice of focusing on the things you appreciate and are thankful for in your life. By actively cultivating an attitude of gratitude, you can shift your perspective from one of scarcity to one of abundance, fostering feelings of contentment and satisfaction.

Numerous studies have demonstrated the benefits of gratitude practice for mental health and well-being. By regularly expressing gratitude for the people, experiences, and blessings in your life, you can enhance your mood, reduce stress, and improve your overall outlook on life.

INNER CHILD WORK: This technique involves reconnecting with and healing emotional wounds of the inner child within you. It's an approach based on the idea that incongruent or negative behaviors we have as an adult stem from childhood experiences that were challenging or even traumatic.

Positive self-talk strategies like internal validation, affirmations, and inner child work can address deep-seated issues from the past and help reshape your present and future.

Now that you know that how you talk to yourself has a profound impact, hopefully it will spark some introspection and any necessary correction. By incorporating positive self-talk practices into your daily routine, you can literally change the landscape of your brain to improve mood, promote flexible thinking, enhance self-confidence, and foster greater overall emotional well-being.

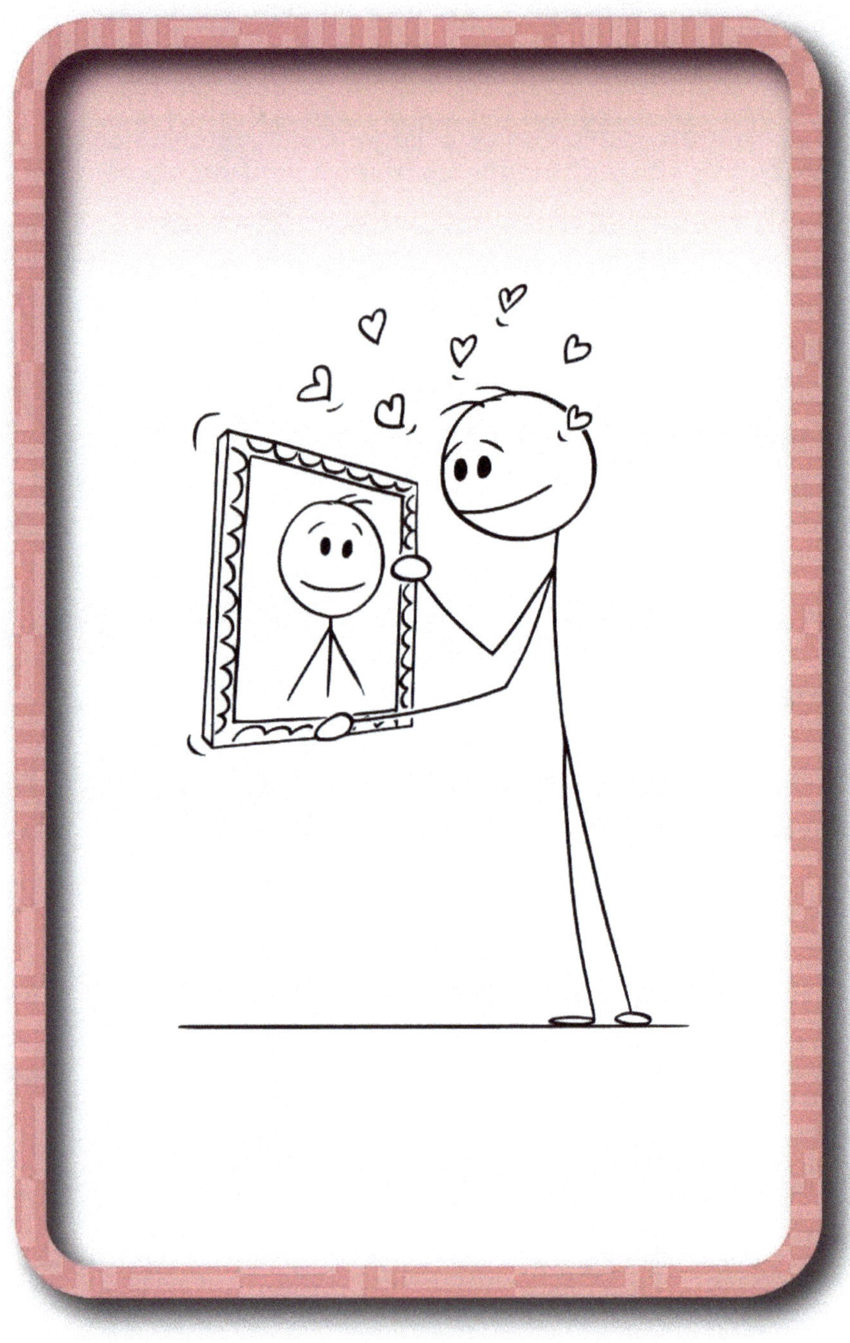

Sample List

Positive Self-Talk

Say daily affirmations

Challenge and replace negative thoughts

Turn off the news

Practice gratitude

Identify wants and needs

Repeat a mantra

Jot down some ideas of your own

____

____

____

____

Chapter 10 Mindfulness

CATEGORY 6: MINDFULNESS

Welcome to the world of mindfulness! In this chapter, we'll dive into the calming sea of present-moment awareness and explore how it can become your trusted companion in navigating life's challenges. OM.

Mindfulness, which is rooted in ancient Buddhist practices, has gracefully made its way into modern psychology as a scientifically researched and proven tool for managing stress, emotional discomfort, and overall mental health. Let's explore the sixth and final category together, discovering mindfulness as an evidence-based practice that holds the potential to transform your life.

What is Mindfulness?

At its core, mindfulness is the practice of being completely present in the moment without judgment. It involves being fully immersed in the here and now, acknowledging thoughts, feelings, sensations, and surroundings with openness and curiosity. While the origins of mindfulness trace back to Buddhist traditions, its adaptation into a modern evidenced-based method has garnered widespread recognition for its effectiveness in reducing mental health symptoms.

Research studies have shown compelling evidence of the benefits of mindfulness practice. For instance, a meta-analysis published in the Journal of the American Medical Association found that mindfulness meditation programs led to small-to-moderate improvements in anxiety, depression, and pain when compared to non-mindfulness interventions. These findings underscore the potential of mindfulness as a valuable coping strategy in today's fast-paced world.

It is said that anxiety is worry about the future and depression is dissatisfaction with the past. Picture this: anxiety as a nagging worrywart always peeking ahead, fretting about what's to come, while depression sits solemnly in the rearview mirror, dwelling on what's already passed. It's like they're the unwelcome backseat drivers of our minds, constantly pulling us away from the present moment. Mindfulness however, is able to keep full attention to "the here and now" keeping calm and taking in the scenery.

Mindfulness isn't about erasing the past or ignoring the future; it's about embracing the present. By tuning into what is happening in the moment (the sights, sounds, and sensations, you can quiet the anxious chatter about what might be and the melancholic rumination about what was.

Practicing Mindfulness

Now, let's take a closer look at some practical applications of mindfulness in coping with everyday stressors and challenges:

Mindful Breathing: One of the most well-known and powerful therapeutic practices is deep breathing. There are many ways to integrate various breathing techniques to benefit mental health. However, in the context of mindfulness, breathing is sometimes referred to as belly breathing or diaphragmatic breathing.

For this simple technique you want to first get comfortable, close your eyes if you wish, and focus on your breath. Then, notice your breath as you inhale and exhale while feeling the rise and fall of your chest. When your mind wanders (as it inevitably will,) gently bring your awareness back to your breathing without judgment. This practice can anchor you to the present moment, promoting a calm state of relaxation and improved mental clarity.

Guided Meditation: This meditation may involve visualization and conducting a body scan. Typically, you are directed to focus on your toes and gradually work your way up to the top of your head, systematically bringing attention to the here and now, noticing any sensations or tension and inviting your body to relax. This practice cultivates body awareness and can help alleviate physical discomfort or tension. There are now many mindful meditation apps on smart devices that can be easily used for guided meditation.

Mindful Walking: You can turn your daily stroll into a mindfulness exercise by paying attention to each step you take. Notice how the ground feels beneath your feet, the swaying of your hands, and the rhythm of your breath. Look around and note the things you can see, hear, smell. Bring your thoughts back to the here and now without getting swept away by thoughts about the past or future. Walking mindfully can be a refreshing way to center yourself amidst the hustle and bustle of daily life.

Mindful Eating: Have you ever mindlessly devoured your meal only to be surprised that you've already finished? Eating while multitasking, like while watching TV, can distract you to the point that you are not paying attention at all. Mindful eating invites you to slow down and use all of your senses for each bite. It includes being aware of the sensations in your mouth and stomach while you eat. If you notice the colors, textures, smells, and flavors of your food, you can have a more satisfying experience. Eating mindfully not only enhances your enjoyment of food but also promotes healthier eating habits and digestion.

Grounding Techniques

In moments of heightened stress or anxiety, grounding techniques can serve as lifelines, helping you reconnect with the present moment and regain a sense of stability. As a type of mindfulness, these techniques can be especially effective in deescalating anxiety or panic attacks. Here are a few grounding exercises to add to your coping toolkit:

5-4-3-2-1 Technique: Engage your senses by identifying five things you can see, four things you can touch, three things you can hear, two things you can smell, and one thing you can taste. This exercise is different than the previously discussed self-soothing techniques since in addition to calming your central nervous system, the intention of this exercise is to anchor you to your immediate surroundings, providing a sense of grounding and safety.

Square Breathing: Visualize a square in your mind's eye. Inhale slowly for four seconds through your nose as you trace one side of the square. Exhale slowly through your mouth for four seconds as you trace the next side. Repeat for the remaining two sides. This breathing pattern will help to calm you and soothe your nervous system.

Grounding Objects: You can discreetly carry a small object with you everywhere you go to use as a grounding tool. Some examples are a furry keychain, a smooth stone, a squishy trinket or a piece of jewelry. When you're feeling overwhelmed, take a moment to hold the object in your hand, focusing on its texture, weight, and temperature. This tangible connection can provide comfort and reassurance in times of distress.

Mindfulness is a skill that most people need to practice, as it does not always come easily. By incorporating mindfulness into your daily life and mastering grounding techniques, you can build resilience in the face of adversity and gain a deeper sense of peace. Remember, the journey of mindfulness is not about perfection but rather about embracing each moment with curiosity and without judgement that can lead to negative feelings.

Dialectical Behavioral Therapy (DBT)

DBT is like the Swiss Army knife of coping strategies, and mindfulness is one of its sharpest tools. Mindfulness, in the context of DBT, isn't about emptying your mind of thoughts or floating off into a Zen-like state. It's about paying attention to what's happening right now, without judgment. Through DBT practices like observing, describing, and participating, you can become more mindful of your internal emotional and physical sensations. This increased self-awareness empowers you to respond to challenging situations with intention rather than reacting impulsively.

Radical Acceptance and Distress Tolerance

I would like to very briefly introduce two very powerful examples of Dialectical Behavior Therapy (DBT) skills: radical acceptance and distress tolerance.

Radical Acceptance: Your life can feel like a high-stakes game of poker, and sometimes, it seems like you're dealt a hand of jokers while everyone else at the table keeps getting aces. Frustrating, right? Instead of stewing in resentment and wishing for a different hand, radical acceptance teaches us to embrace the cards we've been dealt… jokers and all.

Radical acceptance is all about making peace with reality, even when the reality is tough to handle. It's like saying, "You know what? This situation sucks, but it is what it is." It's not about pretending everything's rainbows and unicorns; it's about acknowledging the truth of the moment without adding fuel to the fire of suffering. As Marsha Linehan, the creator of DBT puts it, "Pain is inevitable, but suffering is optional."

Distress Tolerance: Now, let's get back to that poker game. You've got your jokers, everyone else has aces, and you're feeling like the universe's punching bag. Here's where distress tolerance comes into play. Instead of drowning is a sea of rage and consternation, distress tolerance teaches us that we can tolerate discomfort. You have a choice to play your hand to the best of your ability and hope for better cards on the next round or sit there stuck, and suffer wishing that it was different.

DBT teaches when you are caught in the grip of resistance, you might cling to the illusion that things should be different. Radical acceptance and distress tolerance skills are about making a conscious choice to cope rather than crumble. And lucky for you, soon you will have a very handy personalized coping skills toolkit organized into six categories (including mindfulness) to help you cope!

So, the next time life deals you a less-than-perfect hand, remember: radical acceptance and distress tolerance can be your trusty companions in the game of life. Embrace the cards you've been dealt and know that peace lies not in wishing for a different hand, which keeps you stuck in the suffering, but in choosing to cope with the one you've got.

As our last category of coping, mindfulness is a powerful practice centered on being fully present and non-judgmental in the moment. Originating from Buddhist traditions, it has evolved into a widely recognized, evidence-based method for enhancing mental health. Mindfulness helps mitigate the distracting influences of anxiety and depression—those mental "backseat drivers" focused on the future and past—by fostering a calm, present-focused awareness. This approach does not dismiss past or future concerns but rather encourages embracing the present, allowing individuals to quiet their minds and fully engage with their immediate experiences.

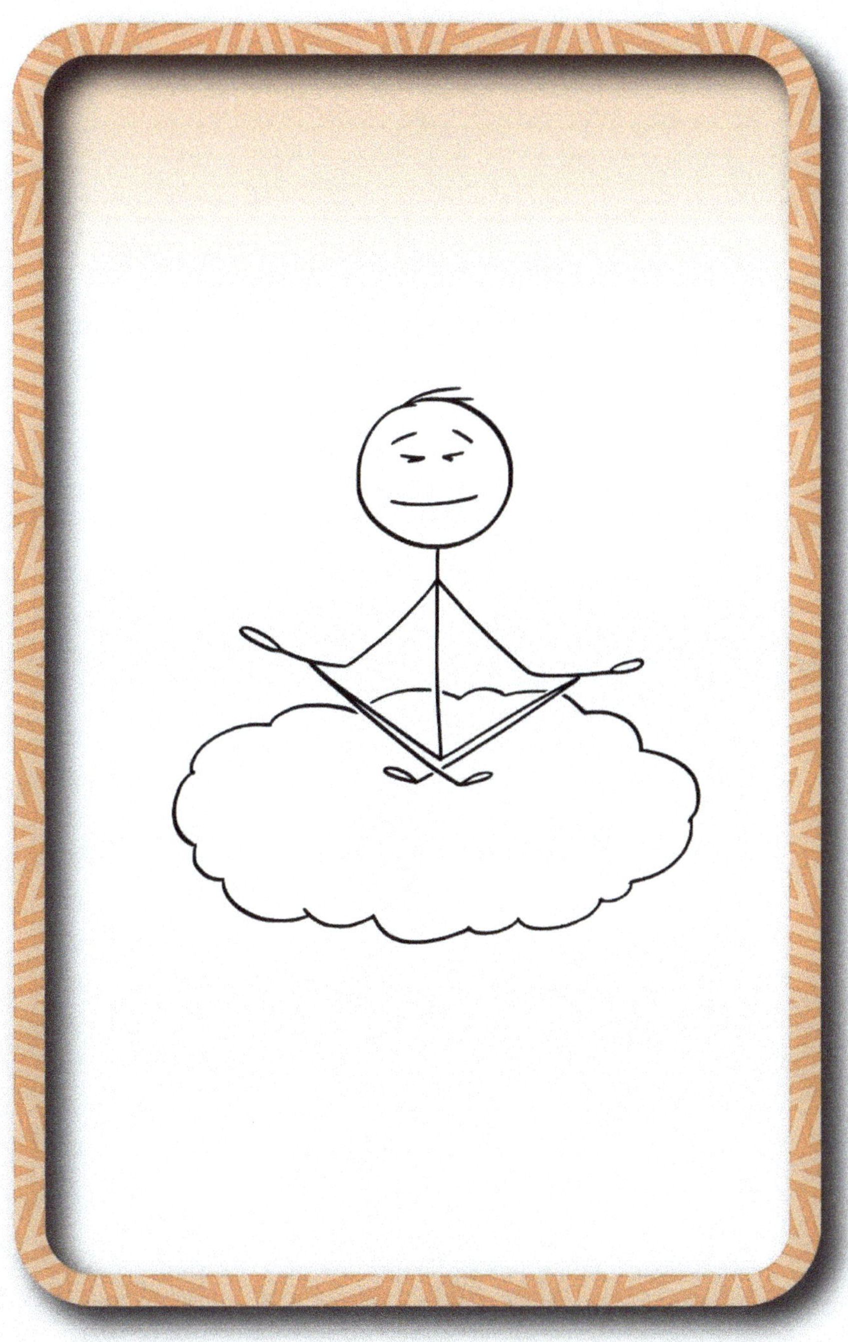

Sample List

Mindfulness

Try meditation

Observe your thoughts without judgement

Go to Yoga class

Bring thoughts back to the present

Use active listening

Turn off electronics

Jot down some ideas of your own

____

____

____

____

____

CONCLUSION

Excellent work! As you reach the final pages of this book, you're stepping into a journey toward preparedness and better self-regulation. You've achieved your goal to create an invaluable and personalized coping skills toolkit to handle life's ups and downs with confidence.

This book isn't just a passive read; it's a dynamic experience designed to empower you in your quest for emotional stability. By categorizing coping skills into six distinct categories, we've laid a solid foundation for you to build upon. From mindfulness and self-soothing techniques to processing and physical strategies, each category offers a wealth of resources to draw from.

In those moments when tension threatens to overwhelm you, remember the power of your customized toolkit. It's your secret weapon against adversity, a source of strength and solace when you need it most. With it by your side, you'll face life's stressors with a plan, knowing that you have the ultimate coping manual at your disposal.

As you glow in the aftermath of accomplishment, remember that the essence of coping lies not just in weathering the storm but in the proactive preparation for it. Your dedication to developing a plan for coping speaks volumes about your commitment to self-care and growth. With each coping skill you add, you reinforce your ability to navigate life's complexities with grace and fortitude. As you move forward, keep in mind that this journey is not about achieving perfection but about embracing progress. Celebrate your victories, no matter how small, and honor the strength within you.

The real magic of this book lies in your very own coping skills toolkit on the next page. Take ownership of your coping journey and continue to add to it over time. As you continue to fill the page with your chosen coping strategies, you're not just creating a toolkit—you're crafting a hack for navigating life's challenges.

So, embrace this book as more than just a guide—it'll be your companion through life's twists and turns. And as you experience hard times, know that you're equipped with everything you need to thrive. Get pumped, and turn the page to review and add to your list!

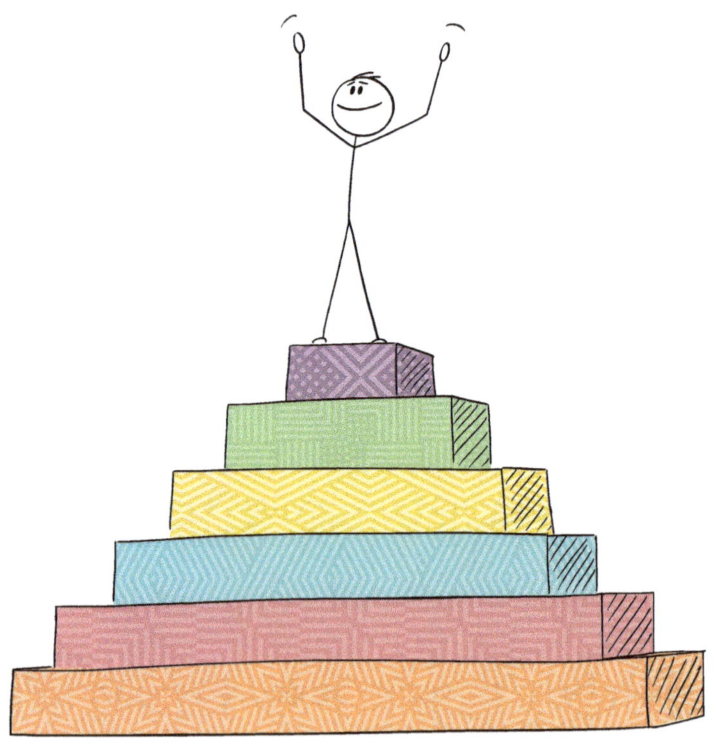

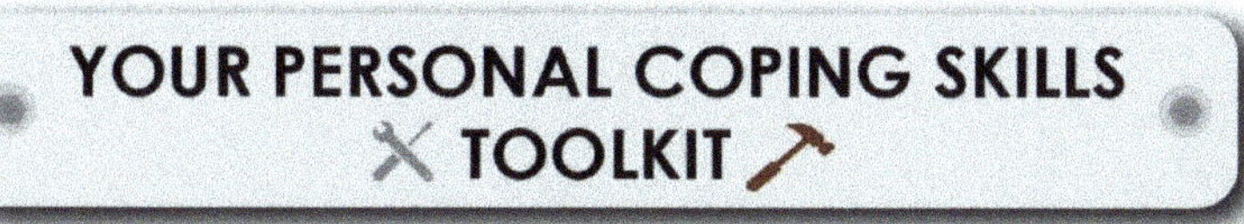

Process	Distract

Self-Soothe	Physical

Positive Self-Talk	Mindfulness

COPING SKILLS IDEAS

Hey there! Welcome to the bonus section of our coping skills book – a handy coping tools menu to help you navigate life's ups and downs like a pro! 🛠️ ✨ Can you think of any coping skills in each category that did not make the list?

In this special section, I've included a list of possible coping skills for each of the six categories which you can use in your own personalized coping skills menu. Since everyone's journey is unique, think of this menu as a springboard for creating and adding to your own customized coping toolkit. Change it up and tweak these coping technique ideas to make them your own!

Watch for the grey flag 🏳️ to indicate the grey area coping skills discussed earlier in the book. This will ensure the coping skills you add to your customized coping skills menu are positive and not used in excess causing negative risk or consequence.

Remember, coping skills are like your trusty sidekicks and they're there to support you through thick and thin. So, explore and let the journey to better well-being begin!

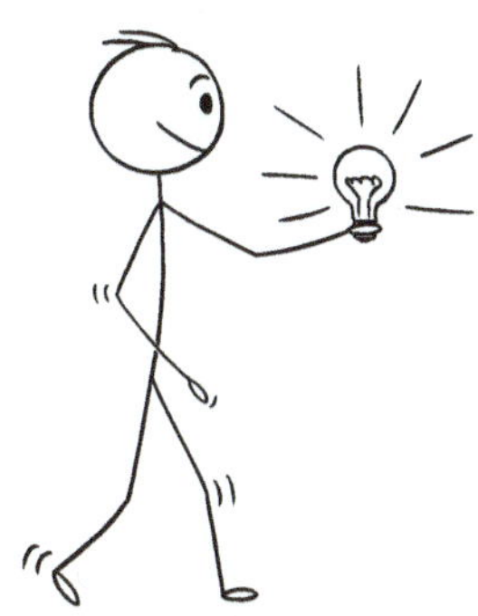

Process

Call a friend

Email your cousin

Weep in your car

Seek support

Share with your clergy

Confide in your brother

Journal your feelings

Send a meaningful meme

Explain it to mom

Jot in your diary

Recount to your dad

Disclose to your therapist

Discuss with your doctor

Go to a support group

Vent to a coworker

Text your sister

See a psychiatrist

Cry with your grandparent

Pray out loud

Join an online forum

Talk to the teacher

Create a checklist

Use "I statements"

Reveal it in a letter

Open up to adult children

Confess to your pet

Brainstorm solutions

Sing about it in the shower

Write about it to a pen pal

Discuss with your plants

Ask for help

Describe it in a poem

Grieve at the grave

Speak to a hotline

Say how you feel

Chat with an aunt or uncle

Whisper to the wind

Feel your feelings

Tell your significant other

Give gratitude

Pinpoint somatic sensations

Set a boundary

Detail a narrative

Express yourself

Communicate your needs

Primal scream

Label the emotion

Distract

Watch TV	Go for a drive
⚑ Scroll your phone	Plan a vacation
See a movie	Clean out a closet
Engage in your hobbies	Try a new physical skill
Read a book	Declutter
Create art	Bake or Cook
⚑ Skim social media	Compile a playlist
Research a topic of interest	Do your hair/makeup
Solve a crossword	Beat a video game
Help someone else	Tidy the house
Laugh at standup comedy	Make a collage/scrapbook
Create a new recipe	Garden or do yardwork
⚑ Take a nap	Redesign your room layout
Walk the dog	Make a craft
Donate to goodwill	Play with the kids
Sort and label your photos	Listen to a podcast
Watch funny videos	⚑ Surf the internet
Complete a puzzle	Fly a kite
Volunteer	Use a fidget
Tackle home improvement	Chat with a friend
⚑ Window shop	Solve a Sudoku
Organize a drawer	Perform car maintenance
Convert home movies	Download memes
	Practice an instrument

Self-Soothe

Put on your PJ's

Cuddle your pet

Drink a cozy beverage

Indulge in dark chocolate

Snuggle up in a blanket

Physical contact

Wear comfy clothes

Take a bubble bath

Swaying or rocking

Chew some gum

Light a scented candle

Listen to white noise

Play calming music

Put on a feel-good playlist

Get a hot shower

Dim the lights

Touch your lips (stimulate parasympathetic fibers)

Splash water on your face

Diffuse essential oils

Bilateral tapping

Swing in a hammock

Practice self-care

ASMR

Cold exposure

Eat a piece of fresh fruit

Get some space

Leave the chaos

Use aromatherapy

Warm in the sun

Change ambient lighting

Get/give a hug

Hug a soft cushion/pillow

6 breaths per minute

Put on scented lotion

Eat something sour

Gargle, hum or sing (to stimulate vagus nerve)

Cold cucumber slices on eyes

Massage your feet

EFT tapping

Go outside/get fresh air

Listen to the rain

Burn some incense

Taste nostalgic flavors

Sit near an open window

Use a weighted blanket

Scalp massage

Physical

Provide adequate nutrition	Use a heating pad
Increase water intake	Workout with a friend
Meal prep for the week	Go swimming
Improve sleep hygiene	Follow medical advice
Light box therapy	Jump rope
Enjoy a funny 80's workout	Go to the gym
Engage in selfcare	⚑ Decrease caffeine
Treat substance abuse	See a Chiropractor
Ride your bike	Consult with a dietician
Take prescribed medication	Unclench your jaw
Progressive Muscle Relaxation	Dance around the house
Get a massage	Find down time to relax
Play a sport	Jog around the block
Go for a walk	Keep a routine
Do some stretching	Get adequate sleep
Exercise at home	Get a facial
Consider acupuncture	Soak in Epsom salt
⚑ Safe consensual sex	Limit processed foods
Reset circadian rhythm	Listen to biofeedback
Focus on healthy eating	Sweat in a sauna
Jump on a trampoline	Squeeze a stress ball
Take a break	Rule out medical causes
Try acupressure	Learn martial arts
Have routine checkups	Schedule a sleep study

Self-Talk

Avoid social media

Use evidence-based practices (CBT, REBT, ACT)

Say affirmations

Reflect on past successes

Acknowledge achievements

Repeat a positive statement

Thought stopping technique

Scroll motivating memes

Take a digital break

Set goals

Embrace radical acceptance

Communicate assertively

Look up inspirational quotes

Self-congratulate

Identify cognitive distortions

Choose a mantra

Question negative thoughts

Approach with humor

Celebrate progress

Have a growth mindset

Catch, check, change intrusive negative thoughts

Implement boundaries

Have self-compassion

Practice gratitude

Read a self-help book

List your best qualities

Explore your values

Reframe your thoughts

Re-read your favorite book

Drop the rope/let go

Reflect on personal growth

Create a daily routine

Forgive

Do inner child work

Be authentic

Don't compare self to others

Build social support

Seek/Ask for help

Visualize success

Increase meaningful activity

Embrace your flaws

Avoid "should" and "must" statements

Let go of perfectionism

Listen to motivating podcast

Turn off the news

Mindfulness

Focus on the here and now

Apply visualization

Relax with guided imagery

Complete a body scan

Sit by a lake

Color a mandala

Knit or crochet

Feel the sand in your toes

Use your senses to explore

Engage in belly breathing

Rake a Zen Garden

Tune into your heartbeat

Create a calming space

Embrace the concept "You are not your thoughts."

Describe what you see

Walk barefoot in the grass

Utilize grounding techniques

Fold origami

Watch running water

Find the constellations

Engage in active listening

Thoughts without judgment

Notice physical sensations

Connect through spirituality

Chant

⚑ Reduce technology use

Sit in silence

Listen to guided meditation

Use a singing bowl

Observe using 5 senses

Apply DBT skills

Notice rhythmic breathing

Meditate

Savor a cup of herbal tea

Practice Yoga

Be in the moment

Name your emotions

⚑ Try mindful eating

Accept thoughts and feelings

Put away distractions

Play binaural beats

Feel textures

Draw or doodle

Do balance exercises

Watch a sunset

Weed the garden

Be one with nature

REFERENCES

Baikie, K. A., & Wilhelm, K. (2005). Emotional and physical health benefits of expressive writing. Advances in Psychiatric Treatment, 11(5), 338–346.Beck, J. S. (2011). Cognitive behavior therapy: Basics and beyond. Guilford Press.

Berntson, G. G., & Bigger Jr, J. T. (2015). The autonomic nervous system and cardiac dynamics. In Handbook of psychophysiology (pp. 279-305). Cambridge University Press.

Cuijpers, P., Karyotaki, E., Weitz, E., Andersson, G., Hollon, S. D., van Straten, A. (2016). The effects of psychotherapies for major depression in adults on remission, recovery and improvement: a meta-analysis. Journal of Affective Disorders, 210, 29-42.

Deci, E. L., & Ryan, R. M. (2000). The" what" and" why" of goal pursuits: Human needs and the self-determination of behavior. Psychological inquiry, 11(4), 227-268.

Ellis, A. (1994). Reason and emotion in psychotherapy: Revised and updated. Citadel Press.

Emmons, R. A., & McCullough, M. E. (2003). Counting blessings versus burdens: an experimental investigation of gratitude and subjective well-being in daily life. Journal of personality and social psychology, 84(2), 377.

Goyal, M., et al. (2014). Meditation Programs for Psychological Stress and Well-being: A Systematic Review and Meta-analysis. JAMA Internal Medicine, 174(3), 357–368. https://doi.org/10.1001/jamainternmed.2013.13018

Grossman, P., Niemann, L., Schmidt, S., & Walach, H. (2004). Mindfulness-based stress reduction and health benefits: A meta-analysis. Journal of Psychosomatic Research, 57(1), 35–43.

Khoury, B., Sharma, M., Rush, S. E., & Fournier, C. (2015). Mindfulness-based stress reduction for healthy individuals: A meta-analysis. Journal of Psychosomatic Research, 78(6), 519–528.

Lieberman, M. D. (2019). Social: Why Our Brains Are Wired to Connect. Broadway Books.

Sherman, D. K., & Cohen, G. L. (2006). The psychology of self-defense: Self-affirmation theory. Advances in experimental social psychology, 38, 183-242.

Thoits, P. A. (2011). Mechanisms Linking Social Ties and Support to Physical and Mental Health. Journal of Health and Social Behavior, 52(2), 145–161.

Van der Kolk, B. A. (2015). The body keeps the score: Brain, mind, and body in the healing of trauma. Penguin Books.

Zucker, T. L., Samuelson, K. W., Muench, F., Greenberg, M. A., & Gevirtz, R. N. (2009). The effects of respiratory sinus arrhythmia biofeedback on heart rate variability and posttraumatic stress disorder symptoms: a pilot study. Applied psychophysiology and biofeedback, 34(2), 135-143.

ABOUT THE AUTHOR

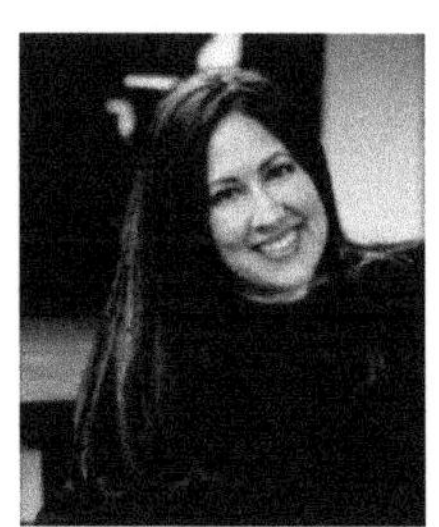

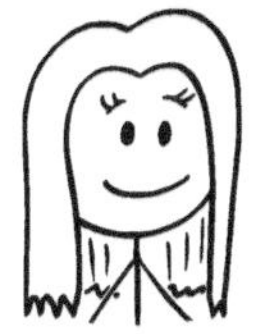

> *Katie Parker MA, LPC is a licensed professional counselor with a mental health career spanning nearly two decades. She has extensive experience working in a variety of clinical settings in various roles. This diverse background has allowed her to gain experience in working with individuals of all ages dealing with concerns ranging from mild issues to severe mental illness. She acts as a clinical mentor, provides trainings to fellow therapists and has been interviewed and published as an authority in the field. Currently, you can find Katie at her private practice Katie Parker Counseling PLLC providing telehealth therapy to adults in Michigan.*

Hi, I'm Katie Parker, MA, LPC. I would like to take a moment to introduce myself and share my mission to transform lives through effective therapy. With a deep commitment to mental health, I have dedicated my career to helping those who are struggling find relief. Working in roles ranging from crisis team member to outpatient therapist, my focus has been helping people to feel better and cope with life's challenges.

Learning positive coping skills and talking through problems are crucial aspects of effective therapy. In addition to incorporating evidence-based methods, I provide psychoeducation to help to enhance wellbeing, reduce mental health symptoms and improve overall quality of life through learning.

Everyday life can be challenging and, at times, utterly overwhelming; you don't have to navigate it alone. It is my hope that this book aligns with the mission to help people find greater peace and happiness. Thank you for letting me be a part of your journey. I wish you excellent mental health!

Congratulations on completing this coping expedition. You're a strong person who has made it through 100% of your bad days! Now, with your customized coping skills toolkit, you can thrive and tackle any challenges that come your way. Great job!

Remember, it may not always be easy, but it is always possible. Happy coping!

For more resources and support from Katie Parker MA, LPC

Visit: katieparkercounseling.com

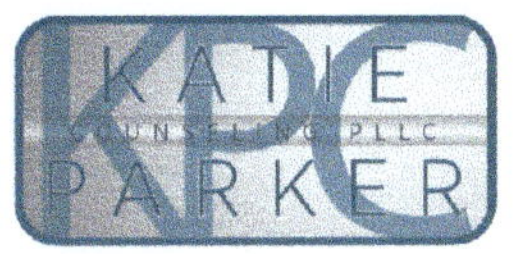

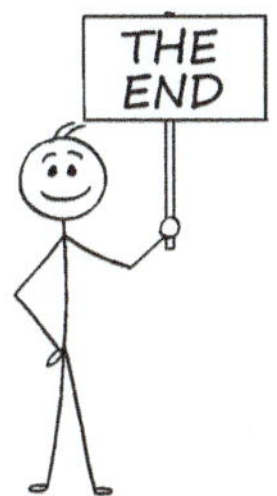